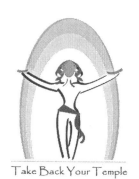

Take Back Your Temple

Take Back Your Temple

Leader Guide

by
Kimberly Taylor

Cover photography by Marcos Santos (http://www.sxc.hu/profile/marcos_bh)
Cover design by Jackie McCutcheon (http://www.jackiemccutcheon.com)

Disclaimer

The information in this guide should be considered as general information only and should not be used to diagnose medical conditions. This guide is sold with the understanding that neither the publisher nor author is engaged in rendering medical advice. The author and publisher shall in no event be held liable for any loss or damages, including but not limited to special, incidental, consequential, or other damages. On any nutrition or exercise plan, individual weight loss results will vary. Your weight loss results will vary based on your starting weight, activity level, and other factors.

Please see your health care provider for diagnosis and treatment of any medical concerns, and before implementing any nutrition, exercise or other lifestyle changes.

Take Back Your Temple Weight Loss Process

A.R.I.S.E.

1. **A**nchor yourself in God
2. **R**enew your Mind
3. **I**nvest in Slimming Foods that Satisfy
4. **S**lim, Stretch and Strengthen your Body
5. **E**xpect Tests and be Prepared

Benefits to expect with practicing the *Take Back Your Temple* process daily:

☑ I am happy about my current size.

☑ I am joyful and excited about life.

☑ I am rarely stressed, worried, or anxious.

☑ I am younger looking than my actual age.

☑ I am focused and make decisions easily.

☑ I am slow to anger, quick to forgive.

☑ I make time to take care of my body every day.

☑ I feel better now than I have in years.

☑ I feel attractive and comfortable in my clothes.

☑ I have a strong faith in God and in my future.

☑ I have loving, close relationships in my life.

☑ I show the love of God to the people I meet.

☑ I have all the energy I need to get my daily tasks done.

☑ I enjoy my food thoroughly.

☑ I regularly eat foods that heal, energize and nourish my body.

☑ I handle negative emotions effectively.

☑ My thoughts are supportive and faith-filled.

☑ I can say no when necessary.

☑ I show grace toward others when under pressure.

☑ I see God's power at work in my life every day.

Measuring Your Progress (*Member Guide pg. 4*)

We recommend measuring fat loss by gauging how your clothes fit and using a tape measure to keep track of inches lost, especially around your waist.

Waist size is an important indicator of your risk in developing diseases such as heart disease, cancer, diabetes, and even Alzheimer's disease. One study showed that stroke risk was **4 times higher** in women with waists above 35 inches and men with waists above 40 inches.

To find your maximum recommended waist size in inches, take your height in inches and divide it by 2. For example, if your height is 5'4" then your maximum waist size should be 32 inches (64 inches ÷ 2). It's recommended that you first focus on improving your health by reducing your waist size, then once successful, set a lower goal for appearance reasons if you like.

- To measure your waist, use the smallest point with your stomach relaxed; if you lack a waist, then measure around your navel.

Optionally, you can also measure your upper arms, bust, hips and thighs. Measure at the widest point and don't "squash" yourself with the tape measure. Every two weeks, re-measure yourself so that you can see your progress.

If you do use a scale to track progress, then use one that shows your weight and your body fat percentage. Even if your weight number may be the same, you may still see your fat % numbers dropping, which is still progress since fat loss is your goal. When you do weigh, do so only every two weeks. Doing so more often may cause anxiety and an unhealthy obsession.

Encourage yourself with other progress signs on your weight loss/greater health plan, including:

☑ Boosted energy
☑ Improved quality of sleep
☑ Enhanced shape and muscle tone
☑ Improved flexibility
☑ Added glow to your skin
☑ Improved endurance
☑ Reduced depression
☑ Improved circulation
☑ Freer breathing
☑ Improved joint discomfort

☑ Increased confidence
☑ Greater mental focus
☑ Increased muscle strength
☑ Better mood control
☑ Enhanced balance and coordination
☑ Increased sexual enjoyment
☑ Increased ability to handle stress
☑ Clearer skin
☑ Increased optimism about life
☑ Amplified desire to tackle other life goals

The above benefits are all signs that you are moving in the right direction! So don't discourage yourself if the numbers aren't moving downward as fast as you'd like. After all, quitting increases the odds to **100%** that you will not get the body and health that you want. Staying on your plan gives you a fighting chance. If you practice the healthy habits recommended, you should consistently lose between 1 - 2 pounds of fat per week, which is a safe rate for weight loss. You will soon look in the mirror and love the results you are seeing!

Dear Friend,

If you are worrying about your weight or your health right now, then I've got a short prayer that can change everything for you as you begin this program and your journey to better health.

A couple of years after God gave me the name "Take Back Your Temple," he gave me its true meaning. Until that point, I always thought of the name as just a challenge to people of faith to take back control of their bodies and their health.

But God told me that I was wrong. "Take Back Your Temple" is a prayer.

This prayer asks God to take control of your body and your life so He can use them for His purpose and agenda. You recognize that you are trying to live in your own strength and *it just isn't working.*

You submit your will to God's will. You recognize that your body is God's temple and you ask Him to guide you in caring for it. You rely on His strength, not your own.

Whatever your struggle, whether it is your weight, destructive habits, or negative emotions like fear, doubt, anger, worry, or depression then simply ask God to: "Take Back Your Temple."

If you pray that simple, powerful four-word prayer with a sincere heart and faith, then it will be answered because it is based on God's own word (1 Corinthians 6:19-20).

Then say "Thank you Lord, I believe that I receive what I've ask for according to Mark 11:24." Repeat this until you feel the joy of receiving the gift bubbling up inside of you.

Expect to feel peace, confidence, and thanksgiving for God's abundant grace (unmerited favor). This is the natural state in which God intends for believers to live.

Now, here is the next step. Many people miss this and so do not obtain what they ask for in prayer. **Listen** as the Holy Spirit speaks to you and guides you, giving you wisdom regarding how to obtain what you asked for in prayer. He is telling you how to transfer what God has already done supernaturally into the natural realm of your experience.

Whatever he tells you to do, do it. Walk out his strategy step-by-step, day-by-day. He will give you the strength you need for today, so receive it by faith.

Don't delay. Each moment you delay is another day that you miss out on the very thing for which you prayed.

May you take this message to heart, apply it in your own life, and forever be blessed in health, healing and wholeness,

Kimberly Taylor
Creator of 'Take Back Your Temple'

Table of Contents

WELCOME – FOR LEADERS...9

GROUP LEADER PREPARATION 11

TIPS FOR CLASS SUCCESS...14

PROGRAM OVERVIEW – FOR MEMBERS 15

ABOUT THE WEEKLY CLASSES 17

WEEK 1: LET US A.R.I.S.E. AND BUILD 21

WEEK 2: A: ANCHOR YOURSELF IN GOD....................................33

WEEK 3: R: RENEW YOUR MIND 45

WEEK 4: I: INVEST IN SLIMMING FOODS THAT SATISFY, PART 1 57

WEEK 5: I: INVEST IN SLIMMING FOODS THAT SATISFY, PART 2 71

WEEK 6: S: SLIM, STRETCH, AND STRENGTHEN YOUR BODY 87

WEEK 8: PUTTING IT ALL TOGETHER 121

APPENDIX 127

Using Food to Balance Your Mood.. *127*
Health Tracking Log - Weekly *129*
Slimming Meal Tips.. *130*
Making Meals Convenient and Delicious *133*
Overcoming Barriers to Exercise... *139*

My Small Group Study

Day we meet:_____   Time we meet:_____

Where we meet:_____

Group leader:_____   Phone number:_____
                                             Email address:_____

Group leader:_____   Phone number:_____
                                             Email address:_____

Note: Any regularly scheduled class that conflicts with a holiday or other special event may be rescheduled.

My Classmates

Name:_____   Phone number:_____
      Email address:_____

Name:_____   Phone number:_____
      Email address:_____

Name:_____   Phone number:_____
      Email address:_____

Name:_____   Phone number:_____
      Email address:_____

Name:_____   Phone number:_____
      Email address:_____

Name:_____   Phone number:_____
      Email address:_____

Name:_____   Phone number:_____
      Email address:_____

Name:_____   Phone number:_____
      Email address:_____

Name:_____   Phone number:_____
      Email address:_____

Name:_____   Phone number:_____
      Email address:_____

Name:_____   Phone number:_____
      Email address:_____

Name:_____   Phone number:_____
      Email address:_____

Welcome – For Leaders

Thank you for your commitment to becoming a *Take Back Your Temple (TBYT)* group leader! TBYT is designed to give members the confidence, knowledge, and skills to reach their best weight and maintain it for life. **It is not about size, but about stewardship – helping others maximize the wonderful body God has given them to manage.** The following is the guiding scripture for the study:

1 Corinthians 6:19-20
Or do you not know that your body is the temple of the Holy Spirit who is in you, whom you have from God, and you are not your own? For you were bought at a price; therefore glorify God in your body and in your spirit, which are God's.

Group leaders are creative and strive to provide effective, practical solutions to help members achieve their ideal weight and maintain it for life. They believe in the benefits of a healthy lifestyle and strive to create a supportive environment so that members can reach their goals more easily.

The following are the ideal characteristics of a *Take Back Your Temple* group leader:

- They love God and love their group members
- They strive to be the change they want to see in others
- They are people of integrity – they "walk their talk"
- They cultivate respectful, supportive relationships
- They are caring and encouraging
- They have a "can-do" spirit
- They are truthful, but tactful
- They are energetic
- They are patient

Important: TBYT Group Leaders may not use their affiliation with TBYT to promote or influence the sale of weight loss supplements, treatments, devices, or professional services.

Being a Learner and a Leader

Understanding group dynamics

Your role is to encourage group interaction, creating a supportive environment. You should not do all the talking but encourage members to share their experience and advice when applicable.

Answering hard questions

While you don't have to know all the answers as a *Take Back Your Temple* group leader, you do need to have the ability to say, "I'm not sure about the answer to that one. Let me research that and I'll have the answer for you by the next class."

Then contact a local health educator, nutritionist, nurse, or other trusted health professional to find an answer. That way, you've learned something new and can pass it on.

Correcting a member tactfully

If a member gives incorrect or incomplete information in class, then give the group the correct information, but give the member credit for those parts of the answer that are correct.

Creating an atmosphere of support and respect

You can feel good knowing that you are bringing the same benefits to members that you have received. If you make members feel important and valued, they will be inspired to value themselves and treat themselves well.

Group Leader Preparation

Tools/Materials Needed

The following materials are needed to teach the course:

For Leaders

- *Take Back Your Temple Leader Guide*
- *Take Back Your Temple Member Guide* (Note: While the *Leader Guide* contains all of the material found in the *Member Guide*, it is helpful to see the material from a member's perspective)
- *Take Back Your Temple Healthy Habits Journal*
- Bible (scriptures in the guides are from the New King James Version)
- Hand weights (for Week 6 demonstration)
- Calculator

For Students

- *Take Back Your Temple Member Guide*
- *Take Back Your Temple Healthy Habits Journal*
- Bible

Leader Notes

Within each week's lesson in the *Leader Guide*, you will see several helpful notes that indicate exercises or suggested discussion questions to engage students in the class.

Depending on student needs or time, you may need to modify the training. Use your best judgment, allowing the Holy Spirit to lead you always.

Preparation for Leaders – 6 Weeks in Advance

A minimum of six weeks in advance:

1. Secure a location to teach the course. Some ideas for locations include churches, libraries, or community centers. Discuss meeting times with the planning committee to determine a time when members can attend.

2. Ask your location contact if at least one other person is available to assist with course implementation (each course should have two leaders).

Before you start Week 1:

1. Read the *Leader Guide* at least once.

2. **Optional:** Contact clinics, hospitals, gyms, and other locations to make a resource list for those in attendance so they will know where they can take exercise classes, or get their blood pressure, blood sugar, or cholesterol checked locally.

   Also contact grocery stores in the area and let them know about the class—they might be able to provide pamphlets, recipe booklets, or other resources to help students implement a healthier lifestyle.

Continued on next page

Preparation for Leaders, continued

At least 1 week before each class:

1. Review the *Leader Guide* two to three times. If you find information you don't understand, ask advice from a trusted health professional.

   To increase confidence, it might help to rehearse your presentation with a friend or family member.

2. Read the instructions for each homework activity.
3. Make a list of tasks you need to do to prepare for class, for example, making adequate copies of the sample food label for students from the Leader Guide for the quiz on label reading in Week 5 or hand weights for the weight training demonstration in Week 6.

Day of the class:

1. Check your task list and ensure that you have all of the materials needed. For example, ensure that you have the copies of the sample food label for students from the Leader Guide for the quiz on label reading in Week 5 or the hand weights for the demonstration in Week 6.

2. Make a copy of your member list so that you can take attendance.

3. Arrive at the location ahead of time so that you can set up the room. Allow 30-60 minutes to prepare.

Tips for Class Success

The following are some tips that can help you ensure the success of your group study:

1. **Pray, Pray, and Pray.** Prayer is a powerful spiritual tool since only God can change hearts and lives. Start the class with prayer and end with prayer. Listen to members' struggles during class and pray for them between classes, asking God to provide the strength and resources they need to overcome.

2. **Get Support.** Ask others to share the leadership responsibilities by helping you plan, distribute materials, and other duties. For larger groups, you may divide the class into smaller groups for discussions, appointing leaders for each group.

3. **Order adequate copies of Member Guides and Journals.** Before starting the course, ensure that members will have their own copies of the materials. We recommend purchasing extra copies for any late registrations. Consider including the price of the materials in the class registration fee if the cost is not underwritten by your organization.

4. **Be prepared with each lesson.** Review each week's lesson in the Member Guide ahead of time so that you can understand the content and lead the discussions with confidence.

5. **Be yourself.** Be open and honest - don't be afraid to share your own struggles and challenges. Members will appreciate you for being real and be encouraged to open up by your example.

6. **Manage class time wisely.** Be sure to respect members' time by starting and ending the class on schedule.

7. **Contact your members.** Reaching out to members outside of class via phone, email, or letter to express appreciation for their attendance is a great way to share how much you care about them, which inspires them to want to do well in practicing the principles outside of class.

8. **Support your pastor.** Ensure that you have the support of your pastor or church leadership before implementing any TBYT program at your church.

Program Overview – For Members

Welcome

The *Take Back Your Temple (TBYT) Member Guide* gives you the confidence, knowledge, and skills you need to reach your best weight and maintain it for life. **It is not about size, but about stewardship – maximizing the awesome body God has given you to manage**. Remember, he owns everything, including your body!

> *1 Corinthians 6:19-20*
> *Or do you not know that your body is the temple of the Holy Spirit who is in you, whom you have from God, and you are not your own? For you were bought at a price; therefore glorify God in your body and in your spirit, which are God's.*

You will discover how to cooperate with the power of the Holy Spirit to live a life rich in health and wholeness so that can fulfill your God-given purpose with vitality, freedom, and energy.

Course Goals

The *TBYT* course teaches you how to:

- Strengthen your relationship with God
- Renew your mind to transform your body and life
- Eat to build a strong, slimmer, and healthier body
- Create a body that is energetic and vibrant
- Plan for obstacles to your health goals and how to overcome them
- Practice good health habits for a lifetime so you can more easily maintain your new size

Course Length

The course lasts for eight weeks. Each session lasts for approximately 2 hours.

About the Weekly Classes

Class Descriptions

Week 1: Let Us A.R.I.S.E. and Build

This lesson helps you determine your wellness vision, obstacles, goals, and gives you an initial goal to start. You also learn about the A.R.I.S.E. process and how practicing it daily helps you to achieve a healthy weight for life.

Week 2: A: Anchor Yourself in God

This week, you learn about the importance of starting your day by anchoring yourself in God through prayer, praise, worship and study of God's word. These foundational steps helps you seek God's wisdom to make wise choices for the day and also assists you in better handling daily stress.

Week 3: R: Renew Your Mind

The bible says that you are transformed when your mind is renewed, and this lesson discusses specific techniques for renewing your mind. One of the reasons most weight loss plans fail is attempting to pile new behaviors on top of an old mindset. However, when your mindset supports your efforts, you are able to create changes that last.

Week 4: I: Invest in Slimming Foods that Satisfy, Part 1

You'll review the best ways to eat to reach your perfect weight and how to avoid overeating in this lesson.

Week 5: I: Invest in Slimming Foods that Satisfy, Part 2

This lesson covers some ideas on how to make healthy eating practical such as how to prepare healthy meals, eating out, and reading nutritional labels.

Continued on next page

Class
Descriptions,
continued

Week 6: S: Slim, Stretch and Strengthen Your Body

This lesson discusses the one technique you can use with any exercise that will accelerate fat loss. You'll also learn ways that you can tone your muscles and stretch your body so that you can perform your daily living activities with greater ease, comfort, and energy.

Week 7: Expect Tests and Be Prepared

In spite of your best intentions, you will be tested and tempted in your desire to reach your perfect weight. This lesson discusses some of the most common obstacles you are likely to face and provides solutions for dealing with them.

Week 8: Putting it All Together

This lesson covers ways that you can maintain good health habits so that once you reach your perfect weight, you are able to maintain it.

*Commitments
You Need to
Make for
Success*

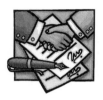

To receive maximum benefit from the Member Guide, commit to the following:

- **Prayer**

  Pray every day for God's protection, provision, wisdom, and courage for yourself and your classmates.

- **Class Attendance**

  To get maximum benefit from the class and to receive your certificate of completion, you must attend six out of the eight sessions. If you are unable to attend a session or you will be late, please notify one of your group leaders in advance to avoid class disruptions.

- **Memory Scripture**

  Memorize the focus scripture each week.

- **Lesson Study**

  Read each lesson and write down any new habits you will adopt.

- **Think About It**

  Complete each day's *'Think About It'* activity. They will help you renew your mind to support your weight loss goals.

- **Walking it Out**

  These action steps are designed to help you get the results you want.

- **Consistent Practice of New Habits**

  A "hit or miss" approach to change yields hit or miss results. Commit to practicing new habits every day for consistent results. Small steps yield big results!

Week 1: Let Us A.R.I.S.E. and Build

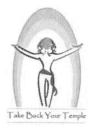

Take Back Your Temple

Week 1 Focus Scripture:

So I answered them, and said to them, "The God of heaven Himself will prosper us; therefore we His servants will arise and build"

- Nehemiah 2:20

Lesson Goals

Member Guide pg. 15

In this lesson, you will learn how to:

- Create your weight loss vision
- Determine your strengths in reaching your vision
- Define obstacles standing in the way
- Evaluate resources to handle the obstacles
- Define the A.R.I.S.E. process

Lesson Agenda
Quick Overview

- Welcome
- *Tense, Breathe, Jello Shake* exercise
- Class Introduction
- Distribute books/materials
- Start Vision Worksheet
- Introduction to the A.R.I.S.E. process
- Homework Assignment

Leader Lesson Agenda

- (5 minutes) *Open in prayer.*
- (10 minutes) *Welcome* – Leaders introduce themselves. For example, share a personal story about your own health struggles and how you came to believe in the importance of health. Keep it light and friendly.
- (5 minutes) *Class Introduction* – Introduce Take Back Your Temple and explain the "It's not about size, but about stewardship" philosophy and what that means to you. Explain why you choose this workshop and why you're passionate about helping others reach their health goals.
- (5 minutes) *Tense, Breathe, Jello Shake* exercise – Lead participants through the exercise to relieve stress and loosen everyone up. You demonstrate first and then ask everyone else to follow along:

   First, everyone stand up. Tense every part of your body, squeezing your hands together into fists at your side. Hold the tension for three seconds.

   Say, "This is the day…"

   Next, inhale and raise your arms to the sky while saying, "That the Lord has made. I will rejoice…."

   Then, exhale and shake your arms down, shaking your hips at the same time like your body is made of Jello while shouting, "And be glad in it!"

   To finish, inhale and exhale with your arms at your sides, feeling deep relaxation.

   Repeat twice.

- (20 minutes) *Distribute the Member Guides and journals* - Ask everyone to turn to pages **7-8 in the Member Guide**, then ask each person to give their names and contact information so that they can complete the information. Also ask them if they could describe themselves positively using one word that starts with the first letter of either their first or last name, what would it be?
- (60 minutes) *Lesson review and discussion* – see each topic for key points.
- (10 minutes) *Review next week's Homework Assignment instructions*
- (5 minutes) *End in prayer.*

Lesson
Introduction

Member Guide
pg. 16

This lesson, *Let Us A.R.I.S.E. and Build*, is about building your health goals on a sure foundation. You create a strong health vision and learn how to transform your vision to reality.

The secret of permanent weight loss is **faith working through love**. Faith arises from knowing God - and the first thing to know is that he loves you. You cannot be motivated to take care of yourself unless you know this first.

When you are convinced of God's love, this is what happens:

1. You draw near to God.
2. God draws near to you and reveals his character and wisdom to you.
3. You increase your faith in God's power and might.
4. You grow in confidence and ability to overcome any challenge that you face, including weight loss challenges.

Next, you need to know these facts (1 Thessalonians 5:23):

- You are a spirit
- You possess a soul (mind, will and emotions)
- You live in a body

Your spirit always wants to do what is right and pleases God. But your body and un-renewed mind are like spoiled children, wanting everything their way. They often compel you to do just what feels good in the moment, whether it is for your ultimate good or not.

So at the beginning of the course, your struggle likely looks like this:

Un-renewed Mind + Body > Spirit

However for the first three weeks of the course, you will gain skills that renew your mind and strengthen your spirit. With the combined forces of a clear vision, stronger spirit, and renewed mind, you can then discipline your body and operate with greater self control.

The battle then shifts in your favor:

Renewed Mind + Spirit > Body

You will then be able to more easily practice the nutritional and exercise guidance that follows in Week 4 and beyond. And you will grow daily in health, healing, and wholeness!

Your Body is a Temple

Member Guide pg. 17

The goal of this course is to empower you to think about your body as a temple and treat it with respect and care. In the bible, the temple was described as:

- Beautiful
- Magnificent
- Glorious
- Great
- Wonderful

When you think of your body in the same terms, then that increases your desire to better care for it. To start taking care of your body, you need a good written plan.

Think of this plan as like one an architect might create before building a house. Planning at the beginning lays the foundation for your future weight loss success.

A good life-changing plan includes:

- Your Vision
- Your Strengths
- Your Obstacles and Plan to Overcome
- Vision Milestones

Your chance of success is much stronger when you write your plans down instead of just relying on memory.

Another important part of your planning is to think about how you can set up a healthy environment in your home to support your goals.

Before we plan your temple's renovation, it will be helpful to review the principles guiding the first temple's construction in the bible.

The process was a sacred one, requiring careful planning and preparation. Let's take a few moments to get some background on that process to renew your mind on the importance of caring for your own body today.

***Member Guide
pg. 18***

***Leader Note:
Ask students to
take turns
reading each of
the scriptures
in this section
aloud, one
scripture per
student until all
of them are
read.***

***Then, ask 1 or
2 students to
explain what
glorifying God
in body and
spirit means to
them according
to 1
Corinthians
6:19-20.***

Here are some scriptures on how King David, the ancient temple planner and King Solomon, the ancient temple builder, viewed the building process:

1 Chronicles 28:10
"Consider now, for the LORD has chosen you to build a temple as a sanctuary. Be strong and do the work."

1 Chronicles 28:20
David also said to Solomon his son, "Be strong and courageous, and do the work. Do not be afraid or discouraged, for the LORD God, my God, is with you. He will not fail you or forsake you until all the work for the service of the temple of the LORD is finished."

2 Chronicles 2:5
"The temple I am going to build will be great, because our God is greater than all other gods."

2 Chronicles 6:2
"I have built a magnificent temple for you, a place for you to dwell forever."

2 Chronicles 6:20
"May your eyes be open toward this temple day and night, this place of which you said you would put your Name there. May you hear the prayer your servant prays toward this place."

And God answered Solomon:

2 Chronicles 7:16
"I have chosen and consecrated this temple so that my Name may be there forever. My eyes and my heart will always be there."

Then in the New Testament comes a special message for you today:

1 Corinthians 6:19-20
"Or do you not know that your body is the temple of the Holy Spirit who is in you, whom you have from God, and you are not your own? For you were bought at a price; therefore glorify God in your body and in your spirit, which are God's."

Your Health Vision

Member Guide pg. 19

Leader Note: *Cover the parts of a health vision on pages 19-20. Students will then create their own for homework using the form on* ***Page 21*** *in the Member Guide.*

The purpose of creating a health vision is to keep you inspired and on track. It helps you mentally make the person you want to be *stronger* than the person that you are now – every day. We'll cover the parts of a health vision then for homework, you'll create your own.

Your health vision is written as if you're already at your desired size. When you do this, you bring the joy of your better future into your present, which gives you motivation to do what is necessary to make it a reality.

The Bible says that God calls those things that do not yet exist as though they did. So to follow His example, you will use present-tense phrases when you write your vision like:

- "I am…"
- "I feel…"
- "I look…"
- "I speak…"
- "I do…"

It is important that you make your vision *present tense*. If you make it future tense, you're communicating that it would be *nice* if you succeed, but it may or may not happen. With present tense, you communicate to yourself *what is happening*.

Make your vision of your future self so real that you feel right now - as you write - all of the feelings that you will experience when you reach that goal like confidence, satisfaction, accomplishment, peace, and joy.

Be sure to include how your body will look and feel and also the positive health habits that you will practice regularly at your perfect size. You want to maintain your new body, right? What health habits will help you age well, keep your mind sharp, and prevent disease?

You can make this vision one page or several pages. The length does not matter, only that it is meaningful and inspiring to you.

Along with your vision of who you want to be, you're going to write why you want to achieve this image. In other words, get clear as to why this is important to you. Your motivation can be positive or negative, depending on which one has the most influence for you. Or you can use both.

For example, you can have a positive motivator, like to become a gorgeous grandmother, or you may have a negative motivator like preventing a disease that runs in your family.

Your Strengths

Member Guide pg. 20

You want to take full advantage of what you already have available to you to assist you in reaching your dream. Some examples of strengths can include:

- God
- Experience
- Creativity
- Time
- Money
- Other people

If you take the time to consider what you already know, then you don't have to start from scratch. Another good resource that you can have is the support of other people. In your own relationships, do you have someone who knows about good nutrition whose knowledge you can use?

Finally, strengthening your relationship with God through regular spiritual practices can help you lower your stress level and stabilize your emotions. If you eat for reasons other than hunger, this will assist you in avoiding using food to handle emotional upsets.

Obstacles and Plan to Overcome Them

When you are working on taking back your temple, you need to consider any roadblocks that might stand in your way. If you don't, then you may stumble in your efforts.

Take a moment to think about obstacles you might face in reducing your size and determine what you are willing to do to overcome the barriers. When you have a plan for handling the obstacles ahead of time, you are more likely to follow through with your plan and less likely to stumble.

Vision Milestones

Everyone has a final goal they want to reach, whether it is a specific size or weight. But it is important that you also establish milestones on the way so that you will know that you are on the right track and can use to encourage yourself.

For example, you might set objective milestones, like celebrating every 2 pounds or every inch lost. Even better, write down subjective milestones, like improvements in how you look and feel. Use the benefits listed at the beginning of the guide for some ideas.

Your Health Vision Worksheet

My Health Vision

_____
_____
_____
_____
_____
_____
_____
_____

My Strengths

_____
_____
_____
_____
_____
_____

My Obstacles and Plan to Overcome Them

_____
_____
_____
_____
_____
_____

Vision Milestones

_____
_____
_____
_____
_____
_____

How I Can Make Staying Healthier Easier for Myself

_____
_____
_____

Overview of the A.R.I.S.E. process

Member Guide pg. 22

Leader Note:
Ask students: "If you met someone who was trying to decide whether to start a program to reach their ideal weight but was feeling discouraged because of previous failures, what would you say to inspire them to try again, plus stick with it until the end?

The A.R.I.S.E. process that you will follow for the rest of the course helps you approach each day strategically so you will achieve your health vision. The first two steps give you the strength, faith, and power to accomplish the last three. These are the missing ingredients in most weight-loss programs and the reason why they fail.

In a typical diet, you attempt to pile new behaviors on top of the old mindset. Eventually, the process starts to feel so uncomfortable that your old mindset convinces you to quit. You eventually end up in the same shape you were before or even worse.

But with this process, you change your mindset and attitude towards caring for your body. This is necessary to keep the weight off permanently.

The word *'arise'* means to:

- get up again
- acknowledge your source
- come to attention

If you've previously fallen down when attempting to lose weight, this is your chance to *get up again.* Secondly, you will acknowledge that you are *putting God first* in all things since He is the source of your life and everything you have. Finally, to *come to attention* means paying attention to your body's needs. You do the things that heal, energize, and strengthen your body to increase your ability to enjoy life.

Here are the five steps of A.R.I.S.E.:

Step	Action
1	**A**nchor yourself in God
2	**R**enew your Mind
3	**I**nvest in Slimming Foods that Satisfy
4	**S**lim, Stretch and Strengthen your Body
5	**E**xpect Tests and be Prepared

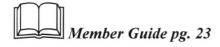 *Member Guide pg. 23*

Step 1: Anchor yourself in God

Because God never changes, anchoring yourself in Him gives you the ideal source to lean on when circumstances seem beyond your control. Your faith helps you during emotionally tough times and gives your life purpose and meaning. So you start your day by connecting to the greatest energy source: a solid relationship with your Creator.

Step 2: Renew your Mind

Step two is critical because your thinking must support your new weight loss habits if you are to continue them long enough to see results. Otherwise, you'll sabotage yourself and quit because your old habits will try to re-assert themselves. But when you renew your mind patiently and consistently according to God's word, you prevent this from happening.

Step 3: Invest in Slimming Foods that Satisfy

With this step, you focus on eating foods that help you drop weight most efficiently, even as they heal, energize, and nourish your body. Plus, you'll maximize your health, improve your mental focus, and bring vitality to your body. Another great benefit is that these foods contain a mother lode of the vitamins and minerals that nourish your skin, giving it a younger, more supple appearance.

Step 4: Slim, Stretch and Strengthen your Body

The fourth step will show you how to burn maximum fat in minimum time. Let's face it – most of us don't have hours and hours to devote to exercise. So you'll learn powerhouse moves that turn your body into a fat-burning furnace. You'll also reshape your body into a shape that pleases you. At the same time, you'll strengthen your heart and find new sources of energy you never knew you had. Soothing stretches will balance your body and help you manage stress better.

Step 5: Expect Tests and be Prepared

Even the best plans can go astray if you aren't prepared for setbacks to your weight loss challenges. This step gives you practical strategies to manage common scenarios that can derail your efforts – such as lack of time, dining out, holidays, emotional eating, and other situations.

As you consistently perform each step, you'll strengthen yourself in mind, body, and spirit as you lose weight. You'll experience new levels of joy and peace.

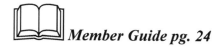 *Member Guide pg. 24*

Week 1 Homework Instructions

Leader Note: Explain the activities for homework to be completed <u>before</u> Week 2's class

Think About It Study:

1. Read 1 Chronicles 28:8-10 and verse 20. What were some of the words of advice that King David passed on to his son, Solomon?

   _____

   _____

2. How can you increase your confidence that you will succeed in taking back your temple?

   _____

   _____

3. Do you have any concerns regarding how you will take back your temple? If so, how can you handle them?

   _____

   _____

4. Read 2 Chronicles 7:12-18. What was God's promise to Solomon in verses 15 and 16?

   _____

   _____

5. In light of God's view of the ancient temple, how does this change your appreciation of your own body?

   _____

   _____

Walk it Out Activity:

- Each week, you will memorize the following week's focus scripture which is at the beginning of each week's lesson.
- Complete your Health Vision Worksheet, using the information about each section in the guide. Don't forget to include your *why*!
- Use your Healthy Habits Journal to write down everything you eat and drink for the week. *If it goes into your mouth, write it down.* This is just part of planning and information gathering; **don't change anything yet.**

Leader Note: Explain other class guidelines below:

- In this class, you will notice that we do not weigh in class; however you can choose to weigh or take measurements to track your progress on your own. Guidelines for measuring your progress are given at the beginning of the Member Guide.
- We do not weigh because we want the focus to be on helping you implement healthy habits for life because if you do that, you will reach your ideal size.
- However, we will **check your health journals each week** to ensure that you are completing them since it is very important that you pay attention to your own health habits so that you can modify them to help you reach your goals.
- **Each day, write down your food intake and any physical activity that you do. Continue through the whole course.**
- Along with checking your health journals, we will have discussions about what you are learning from journaling your health habits, so again it is important that you are faithful with keeping your journal.

Week 2: A: Anchor Yourself in God

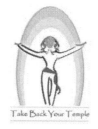

Take Back Your Temple

Week 2 Focus Scripture:

Through wisdom a house is built,
And by understanding it is established;
By knowledge the rooms are filled
With all precious and pleasant riches.

- Proverbs 24:3-4 (NKJV)

Lesson Goals

*Member Guide
pg. 25*

In this lesson, you will learn how to:

- Ask God for help with your health goals
- Study to strengthen yourself in God's word
- Pray for God's will
- Speak to move the mountains in your life
- Walk out the will of God
- Exercise patience for your vision to come to pass
- Translate your new spiritual commitment into physical action

*Lesson
Agenda*

*Quick
Overview*

- Welcome
- *Tense, Breathe, Jello Shake* exercise
- Recite this week's focus scripture
- Review the previous week's homework
- Review this week's lesson
- Homework Assignment

Leader Lesson Agenda

- (5 minutes) _Open in prayer._
- (5 minutes) _Tense, Breathe, Jello Shake exercise._
- (5 minutes) _Welcome everyone to class and document attendance._
- (10 minutes) _Ask each person to recite this week's focus scripture._
- (20 minutes) _Review the previous week's homework – answers follow on the next page._
- (10 minutes) _Journal review_ – Ask each person to turn in their Healthy Habits journals for review.

Ask the class to divide themselves into groups of 2 or 3. While you are reviewing the journals, ask each group to discuss the following question: _"In keeping your journal, what healthy habits did you discover you are already practicing? Which habits would you like to change?_

After you have checked the journals, return them to their owners.

- (50 minutes) _Review this week's lesson and discuss_
- (10 minutes) Homework Assignment instructions
- (5 minutes) _Close in prayer and ask students for specific prayer needs/requests._

Week 1 Homework – Answers

Leader Note: Have homework group discussion, asking for feedback for each question.

Think About It Study:

1. Read 1 Chronicles 28:8-10 and verse 20. What were some of the words of advice that King David passed on to his son, Solomon?

    Know the God of your father, and serve Him with a loyal heart and with a willing mind; If you seek Him, He will be found by you; Consider now, for the LORD has chosen you to build a house for the sanctuary; be strong, and do it."

2. How can you increase your confidence that you will succeed in taking back your temple?

    - *Ask 1-2 students to contribute to this discussion.*

3. Do you have any concerns regarding how you will take back your temple? If so, how can you handle them?

    - *Ask 1-2 students to contribute to this discussion.*

4. Read 2 Chronicles 7:12-18. What was God's promise to Solomon in verses 15 and 16?

    God's eyes will be open and ears attentive to prayer made in His temple. He chose and sanctified his house that His name may be there forever; and His eyes and His heart will be in his temple forever.

5. In light of God's view of the ancient temple, how does this change your appreciation of your own body?

    - *Ask 1-2 students to contribute to this discussion.*

Lesson
Introduction

Member Guide
pg. 26

Picture a ship, rocking and rolling as it tries to navigate stormy seas. Each wave threatens to take it down. The poor ship is at the mercy of the waves rising against it.

Now imagine that same ship in a harbor, anchored securely. Storms may come, but the ship is in a place where it is protected and safe.

That is what anchoring yourself in God is like. You will have troubles in life, but you are confident that you will weather them—all because God is present with you. So you must spend time with God every day.

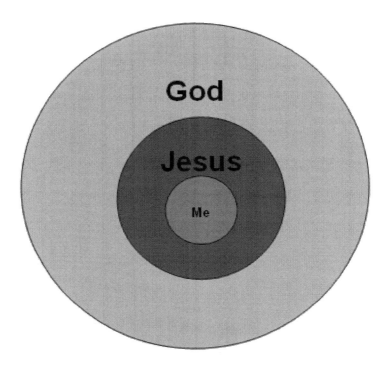

This lesson will teach you how to strengthen your personal relationship with God so that you can stand strong through any challenges that come your way, whether through the weight loss process or through other areas of your life.

Wisdom,
Understanding
and Knowledge

Member Guide
pg. 27

Three benefits are yours through anchoring yourself in God: wisdom, understanding, and knowledge. *Wisdom* is the foundation of your life. It starts with having security in your identity in Christ through salvation.

Understanding is the revelation of the Holy Spirit and is comparable of the support beams and roof of the house. The Holy Spirit instructs you on what to let into your house and what to keep out. His guidance is sure; He is **never** wrong.

Finally, *Knowledge* is the knowledge of God and Jesus Christ that fills your house. This relationship gives your life richness and is the key to abundant life. In fact, it is **the** secret to life. Everything else is secondary.

Now let's look at 7 practical steps on how you can anchor yourself in God each and every day. The more you do these steps, the more God's power will be released in you, which will enable Him to do amazing things in your life.

These steps are:

- Ask
- Study
- Pray
- Speak
- Do
- Wait
- Watch

Ask

One of the first things to ask of God is *wisdom*. To succeed with your weight loss goals, you need the ability to judge correctly and follow the best course of action.

As you grow in wisdom, you will begin to make choices between temporary pleasures versus those that have lasting value, like your health. You will find it becoming easier to invest in your health with each passing day. As you make more investments in your health through eating well and regular physical activity, you will get an abundant return with exploding energy and the ability to enjoy a body that pleases you.

Secondly, ask God for hunger to study His word and additional wisdom to apply it to your daily life. Seeking God's will for your daily life will not only help alleviate the daily stress that contributes to destructive habits, but can likely head off some problems before they even start!

Leader Note:
Ask students to take turns reading the encouraging scriptures in this section, one scripture per student.

Commit to studying the word of God to discover what God says about health and healing. This is so important to giving you strength and encouragement.

Here are a few scriptures to encourage you. You might also want to copy each scripture on an index card and review the cards throughout the day to refresh your mind and spirit.

Romans 14:17
"…for the kingdom of God is not eating and drinking, but righteousness and peace and joy in the Holy Spirit."

2 Corinthians 5:17
"Therefore if anyone is in Christ, he is a new creature; the old things passed away; behold, new things have come."

Philippians 1:6
"For I am confident of this very thing, that He who began a good work in you will perfect it until the day of Christ Jesus."

Hebrews 12:11
"All discipline for the moment seems not to be joyful, but sorrowful; yet to those who have been trained by it, afterwards it yields the peaceful fruit of righteousness."

3 John 1:2
"Beloved, I pray that in all respects you may prosper and be in good health, just as your soul prospers."

Reading the word, especially aloud, is a great form of studying, but it's not the only one. You can also listen to the bible on audio or you can even watch spiritual sermons on video, television, or the Internet.

Your ultimate goal is to allow God's word to have a greater impact on your life than the influence of the world. It's an incredible way to experience more of God's goodness in your life.

Pray

Member Guide
pg. 29

It is recommended that you start a habit of morning prayer time to anchor yourself in God and seek his help to start your day. The more time you are able to spend with him, the more benefits you will gain. Let prayer be your **first** defense against the challenges of life!

During your prayer time, actively seek for God's will to be done in your daily life. In your weight loss journey, it will be much easier to make wise decisions in an atmosphere of peace and no place is more peaceful than in the center of God's will for you.

You also want to fervently pray God's word back to Him. As you do so, you are assured that you are lining up your will with His. You can also be confident that God watches over His word that He may perform it.

In addition, pray when you feel anxious about **anything**. You might know that children are taught they should "Stop, Drop & Roll" if their clothes catch on fire.

In like manner, when your life is on fire and any situation concerns you, great or small, your automatic reaction should be to "Stop, Drop & Pray."

In other words, take a moment to acknowledge the negative emotion you are feeling (stop), humbly acknowledge your need for God (drop), and ask God for help in your situation (pray).

You can "Stop, Drop & Pray" anytime and anywhere. The "Drop" does not mean you need to get on your knees or even lower your head or eyelids. Instead, it is a position of the heart. In humility, you recognize God's power and your total dependence on Him to get you through life.

Philippians 4:6-7 gives this prescription for anxiety:

Be anxious for nothing, but in everything by prayer and supplication, with thanksgiving, let your requests be made known to God; and the peace of God, which surpasses all understanding, will guard your hearts and minds through Christ Jesus.

So be anxious for nothing, but pray about everything...with thanksgiving!

As a believer, you can go to God with boldness and thanksgiving. Take advantage of this incredible privilege so that you can live a life that glorifies God.

Leader Note:
*Ask students to
read the
positive bullet
points in this
section aloud
in unison –
with energy
and
enthusiasm.
Ask them how
they feel
afterwards.*

When you speak God's word out loud, you will feel even more power and strength. According to the bible, faith comes by hearing and hearing by the word of God. To prove this to yourself, take note of how you feel now; then read the following statements with as much energy as you can:

- "I prosper and am living in health as my soul prospers."

- "I praise God because I am fearfully and wonderfully made. Marvelous are His works and that my soul knows very well."

- "I bless the Lord and remember all His benefits. He forgives all of my sins. He heals all of my diseases."

- "I can do all things through Christ who strengthens me."

- "I am anxious about nothing but I pray about everything."

Now close your eyes for a moment. Do you feel a renewed sense of peace and confidence? That is the power of faith that will help sustain you during more challenging times. Even if you aren't happy about your current size right now, you can still experience God's peace and confidence in the midst of it when you speak His promises over your life.

That way, you can enjoy the process of *Take Back Your Temple* as it happens, instead of saving your joy for the day when you reach your ideal size.

Do

As you study the word of God, you will learn more about His character and will. The bible is the ultimate source of wisdom. In fact, the book of Proverbs is solely devoted to living a successful daily life rich in God's wisdom. It is easy to allow your feelings to control you if your sole source of wisdom is from the world. Only God's wisdom will allow you to take the best course of action so that your feelings take a backseat to your faith.

As you faithfully act in accordance with God's will for your life you will discover new sources of strength and joy.

Wait

Member Guide
pg. 31

Our culture is trained to want results yesterday! But in God's system, He has a definite purpose in the wait. His word says:

James 1:4
But let patience have its perfect work, that you may be perfect and complete, lacking nothing.

God works all things out for your ultimate good so that you will lack nothing. Have confidence that each day is a fresh opportunity to strengthen yourself in God and to get another step closer to reaching your ideal size.

Focus on making deliberate, meaningful steps toward good health, knowing that as you do so, your results will appear in time.

Continue to ask, study, pray, speak, and do the will of God diligently every day.

For added power in your wait, be sure to praise God in advance for what He is doing in your life now and what He will do in the future. This will give you a new perspective and will make the wait seem much shorter!

Watch

Each day, take note of the changes that are taking place, spiritually, mentally, emotionally, and physically. You will feel lighter in body and less stressed in mind. Expect that God will perform His word as He said he would.

As you anchor yourself in God, you will see more evidence of the fruit of the Spirit that is promised to us as believers: You will experience more love, more joy, patience, kindness, goodness, faithfulness, gentleness, and self-control. The most exciting thing is that you will see His blessings poured out over your life in a measure that will astound you!

Drinking water is a great reminder of your constant need for God. You can't say, "Well I drank water yesterday so I should be fine today." No, you need a constant supply of fresh water to function at your best. And so you need God in the same way:

John 7:38
He who believes in Me, as the Scripture has said, out of his belly will flow rivers of living water."

Jeremiah 2:13
"For My people have committed two evils: They have forsaken Me, the fountain of living waters, And hewn themselves cisterns—broken cisterns that can hold no water."

As a reminder of the importance of renewing yourself in the spiritual and physical, the first physical habit you'll work on is starting a habit of drinking the recommended amount of water for your body every day.

Think of the difference between a plum and a prune. Plums are firm, juicy and smooth. Prunes are shriveled, dry and wrinkled. A prune is a plum with all the water removed.

It's estimated that 75% of Americans are dehydrated – low water levels in their bodies. Your body is 60-75% water and you lose up to 10 cups of it every day through urination, sweating, and even breathing.

You need water to help you think clearly, to remember (your brain is about 80% water), to cushion your joints and protect them against injury, to use food for energy, eliminate waste, and to maintain a healthy weight.

On the following page, you'll receive some tips on how to maintain the best water levels for your body.

How much water do you need? Most people need a minimum of 8 *cups* per day, however the more you weigh, the more water your body needs. A cup is about 8 ounces, which is smaller than you might think.

Note: If you have kidney problems, bladder control problems, or your doctor has recommended a water restriction for medical reasons, do **not** use these guidelines. Instead, follow your doctor's advice as to how much water to drink each day.

Leader Note: *Ask students to look at the chart that outlines how much water is recommended for their body weight. Ask them to circle the amount that is right for them.*

Use the following guideline for the water amount to drink each day:

Weight	Water Amount
Up to 143 lbs.	8 cups of water per day
144 to 159 lbs.	9 cups of water per day
160 to 175 lbs.	10 cups of water per day
176 to 191 lbs.	11 cups of water per day
Over 191 lbs.	12 cups of water per day

If you currently do not drink this much then simply add an extra cup each day until you reach your recommended amount – then stay there each day.

You can add lemon or lime juice, or use a water filter to help you increase your intake of water. For variety, try drinking herbal teas as well, like chamomile, cinnamon, peppermint, or green teas. You can also make drink fruit juice spritzers as well for variety. Fruit juice is very high in calories, so you want to dilute it whenever possible.

By the way, substituting diet sodas for regular sodas is **not** recommended. According to a recent study, a link exists between drinking diet soda and increased risk of developing metabolic syndrome. This syndrome is a collection of risk factors which include increased belly fat, high blood pressure, and high blood sugar, which are associated with increased risk of heart disease and diabetes.

Pure water is best. Caffeinated beverages and alcohol dehydrates your body. Drinking sugared beverages makes your blood syrupy and eating excess salt makes your blood like the Dead Sea. Both of these make your heart have to pump harder to get the blood flowing, which contributes to high blood pressure and joint pain. If you do eat food high in these substances, be sure to drink a glass of water 1/2 hour before and 1/2 hour after to help dilute your blood so it can flow freely.

Finally, avoid drinking more than 16 ounces per hour to prevent water intoxication; instead drink water regularly throughout the day.

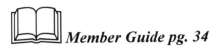

Week 2 Homework Instructions

📄 **Leader Note:** *Explain the activities for homework to be completed <u>before</u> Week 3's class*

Think About It Study:

1. Read 2 Chronicles 20:1-30. In verse 4, how did Judah handle the problem they faced?

   _____

   _____

2. In verses 5-12, what did King Jehoshaphat tell God about Himself?

   _____

   _____

3. In verses 14-17, how did God respond to King Jehoshaphat?

   _____

   _____

4. After God gave Judah the victory, what did the people do to celebrate (see verses 25-30)?

   _____

   _____

5. Write down a situation in which God gave you the victory. What happened?

   _____

   _____

Walk it Out Activities:

- Memorize next week's focus scripture.
- Begin spending time with God in prayer first thing in the morning, asking for wisdom and strength to make wise health choices for that day. Whenever you feel anxious about anything, stop immediately and pray. Expect God to answer your prayer.
- **The Water Challenge:** Read the 'Water Advice' segment and discover how many cups of water are best for you. Next, study your food journal from last week. How many cups of water on average did you drink each day? Add one cup each day until you reach the amount that is best for your body. Record the amounts you drink in your journal. Continue to record your food intake as well.

Week 3: R: Renew Your Mind

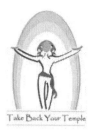

Take Back Your Temple

Week 3 Focus Scripture:

And do not be conformed to this world, but be transformed by the renewing of your mind, that you may prove what is that good and acceptable and perfect will of God.

- Romans 12:2 (NKJV)

Lesson Goals

Member Guide pg. 35

In this lesson, you will learn how to:

- Keep yourself motivated
- Speak your vision to increase inspiration
- Overcome limiting beliefs
- See your vision as already accomplished
- Translate your renewed mind into physical action

Lesson Agenda

Quick Overview

- Welcome
- *Tense, Breathe, Jello Shake* exercise
- Recite this week's focus scripture
- Review the previous week's homework
- Review this week's lesson
- Homework Assignment

Leader Lesson Agenda

- (5 minutes) *Open in prayer.*
- (5 minutes) *Tense, Breathe, Jello Shake exercise.*
- (5 minutes) *Welcome everyone to class and document attendance.*
- (10 minutes) *Ask each person to recite this week's focus scripture.*
- (20 minutes) *Review the previous week's homework – answers follow on the next page.*
- (10 minutes) *Journal review* – Ask each person to turn in their Healthy Habits journals for review.

Ask the class to divide themselves into groups of 2 or 3. While you are reviewing the journals, ask each group to discuss the following question: *"What methods did you find most helpful to establish your water habit this week?"*

After you have checked the journals, return them to their owners.

- (50 minutes) *Review this week's lesson and discuss*
- (10 minutes) Homework Assignment instruction
- (5 minutes) *Close in prayer and ask students for specific prayer needs/requests.*

Week 2 Homework - Answers

Leader Note: Have homework group discussion, asking for feedback for each question.

Think About It Study:

1. Read 2 Chronicles 20:1-30. In verse 4, how did Judah handle the problem they faced?

   So Judah gathered together to ask help from the LORD; and from all the cities of Judah they came to seek the LORD.

2. In verses 5-12, what did King Jehoshaphat tell God about Himself?

   Are You not God in heaven; Do You not rule over all the kingdoms of the nations, and in Your hand is there not power and might, so that no one is able to withstand You? Are You not our God, who drove out the inhabitants of this land before Your people Israel, and gave it to the descendants of Abraham Your friend forever?...For we have no power against this great multitude that is coming against us; nor do we know what to do, but our eyes are upon You."

3. In verses 14-17, how did God respond to King Jehoshaphat?

   "'Do not be afraid nor dismayed because of this great multitude, for the battle is not yours, but God's. ...You will not need to fight in this battle. Position yourselves, stand still and see the salvation of the LORD, who is with you.' Do not fear or be dismayed; tomorrow go out against them, for the LORD is with you."

4. After God gave Judah the victory, what did the people do to celebrate (see verses 25-30)?

   They blessed the LORD; therefore the name of that place was called The Valley of Berachah until this day. Then they returned to go back to Jerusalem with joy, for the LORD had made them rejoice over their enemies. So they came to Jerusalem, with stringed instruments and harps and trumpets, to the house of the LORD."

5. Write down a situation in which God gave you the victory. What happened?

   - *Ask 1-2 students to contribute to this discussion.*

You've probably experienced how uncomfortable change can feel. Whenever you're reaching for any goal, there is always tension between the person you are now and the person you want to be.

The fact is, your mind doesn't like change because its main job is to keep you alive and safe – unfortunately, it often does that by persuading you to keep the habits that you already have. Even though logically you may know that some of your health habits aren't safe, you've done them for so long that your mind thinks they are. So it makes it very uncomfortable for you to change.

It is very well acquainted with you and knows exactly what thoughts will get you to quit your program or to forget how important reaching your ideal size is to you.

Your mind can compel you to do what seems *easiest* in the moment—instead of doing what is *best* for your future.

As you go through *Take Back Your Temple*, you will discover a startling truth: the mental work that you do will be much more challenging than any physical work you will do.

Renewing your mind is about meditating on things that you want to happen. All of the strategies you'll learn this week will show you how to renew your mind so you can be changed both mentally and physically.

The more diligent you are about renewing your mind, the easier it will be to practice the eating and physical activity advice that comes later. And the more consistent you are about practicing the suggestions, the faster your results will come.

Every minute you spend renewing your mind will pay off in the hours you would otherwise spend creating habits that keep you from enjoying physical health and vitality.

Let's review five strategies that you can practice to renew your mind.

Strategy 1: Bring your better future into the present

Member Guide pg. 37

To stay inspired, every day you must mentally make the person you *want to be* stronger than the person that you are now.

In the first week, you created your health vision and were advised to review it regularly. Now, you're going to live this vision— right now! During the day, you will walk as if you're already the size you want to be, and you'll talk as if you're already that size.

Remember this phrase: "If you can't see it, you can't be it." So visualize yourself as already successful and affirm that vision several times each day.

You must do this with all diligence because this brings the joy of your better future into your present. After all, why wait to enjoy your better body? If you start enjoying it now, then you will have an additional motivation to do what you need in order to make it a reality.

Strategy 2: Affirm your vision in your own voice

Leader Note:
Ask students to read the positive bullet points in this section aloud in unison.

A powerful definition of integrity is that "you are the person you say that you are." The question is: "What are you saying you are?" Be sure that the names you call yourself are ones you want to answer to!

Regularly speak your vision out loud in your own voice and see yourself as if you have already achieved it. In addition, speak statements about yourself that are in line with God's word:

- *I am created in the image of God and I praise Him.*

- *I am fearfully and wonderfully made.*

- *I love myself. I accept myself. I value myself.*

- *My body is the temple of the Holy Spirit. Because God's spirit lives in me, I have infinite wisdom available to me.*

- *I use this wisdom to love and care for myself. If I am to live according to God's purpose, my mind, body, and spirit must be strong and healthy. I declare they are so.*

- *God can do exceedingly, abundantly, above all that I can ask or think according to the power that works in me. I invite Him to demonstrate His power in my life today*

Strategy 3: Identify Limiting Beliefs

As you affirm your vision then watch out for negative thoughts that argue with you and tell you that you can't do it.

These are limiting beliefs that need to be dealt with. They can potentially sabotage you while you're taking the actions necessary to reach your new size.

Member Guide pg. 38

Pray for these limiting beliefs to be removed from your mind immediately. Consciously relax your body and challenge these limiting beliefs until the doubts in your mind are gone. When you can say these beliefs without feeling tension in your body and without the doubts arising in your mind, you will feel the power your vision creates in your body.

Strategy 4: Replace Limiting Beliefs with the Truth

Limiting beliefs can arise at any time, not just when you are affirming your vision. So one of your most important skills when losing weight is learning how to replace lies with the truth. Lies like "This is too hard" make you want to give up and quit; but you can prevent this from happening.

Each day, assess your thoughts for limiting beliefs, then replace each one with truth from God's word. You can either do it mentally, or for insistent negative thoughts, speak God's word aloud. Your thoughts must always yield to your spoken word.

God's word is your greatest weapon, but if you don't use it, then you are at the mercy of your old ways of thinking and acting. This leads you away from where you want to be.

Andrew Carnegie, the great steel magnate of the eighteenth century said the following: "The man who develops the ability to control his own mind may then take possession of anything else to which he is justly entitled."

In the Bible, we are told to take our thoughts captive to the obedience of Jesus Christ. But there is no way that we can do that through human effort and thinking. Only God's word is strong enough to overcome the influence of this world. With your bible, you have the power to overcome limiting beliefs and when you use it, you will reap magnificent benefits.

The following is a handy replacement table for some of the most common limiting beliefs regarding weight loss and the scriptures from the bible that challenges them with the truth.

📋 *Leader Note: Ask students to refer to the table on **Page 39** in the Member Guide. Divide the class in half – one half will role-play those who hold limiting beliefs and one half will role-play those who speak God's truth.*

Ask the group who are playing the role of 'limiting beliefs' to say the first belief in unison, in the most discouraging, nasty, whiny, depressing voice ever. The 'God's Truth' group will answer back in a confident, faith-filled, joyful voice. Have them go down the list with each belief.

Then ask the groups to switch so that the 'limiting beliefs' group now becomes the 'God's truth' group and vice versa. Afterwards, ask the class their thoughts on playing each role.

Limiting Belief	God's Truth
"This is too hard."	"I can do all things through Christ who strengthens me." (Philippians 4:13)
"I might as well quit" or "This is taking too long."	"…let us run with endurance the race that is set before us, looking unto Jesus, the author and finisher of *our* faith…" (Hebrews 12:1-2)
"I don't have any self discipline."	"But the fruit of the Spirit is love, joy, peace, patience, kindness, goodness, faithfulness, gentleness and self control." (Galatians 5:22-23)
"I am just meant to stay this way."	"Or do you not know that your body is the Temple of the Holy Spirit whom you have from God and you are not your own but you were bought with a price. Therefore glorify God in your body and in your spirit which are God's." (1 Corinthians 6:19-20)
"I hate my body."	"I will praise You, for I am fearfully and wonderfully made; Marvelous are Your works, And that my soul knows very well." (Psalm 139:14)
"I'd kill for a cookie" or "I'm dying for some pie." (or any other food weakness)	"All things are lawful for me, but all things are not helpful. All things are lawful for me, but I will not be brought under the power of any." (1 Corinthians 6:12) "I shall not die, but live, And declare the works of the LORD." (Psalm 118:17)
"This temptation is too strong. I might as well give in."	"No temptation has overtaken you except such as is common to man; but God is faithful, who will not allow you to be tempted beyond what you are able, but with the temptation will also make the way of escape, that you may be able to bear it. (1 Corinthians 10: 13)

In addition to the previous limiting beliefs, there may be some mental attitudes you need to change. For example, if you've been an emotional eater, then you might think that you need food to manage your emotions.

That is not true. Whenever you feel distressed, your new thinking will be to go to God first. A good scripture to remember with this thought pattern is *Romans 14: 17: For the kingdom of God is not eating and drinking but righteousness, peace and joy in the Holy Spirit.*

A prime cause of emotional eating is holding on to destructive emotions. These emotions can halt your progress and need to be released if you are to move forward in your weight loss process:

- If you are habitually angry, let it go.
- If you are prideful, let it go.
- If you are resentful, let it go.
- If you're jealous, let it go
- If you are envious, let it go.
- If you're unforgiving, let it go.
- If you're bitter, let it go.

As a person of faith, one of the greatest lessons to learn is that *your life is not your own.* Once you accept Christ, you recognize that Jesus bought you at a very high price – his sinless life. So you give up your "right" to the things that you used to do.

Jesus promised that he would send His disciples a helper after His return to the Father in heaven. That same Holy Spirit lives inside of each believer in Jesus today - empowering us to live God's way.

The bible says that if you abide in Him and His word abides in you, you may ask for what you desire, and it will be done for you (John 15:7), according to His perfect will. So ask God for the power to do those things that seem impossible in your human mind. Then hang on and watch Him do the impossible!

On the following page, you'll receive some tips on how to renew your mind to eating mindfully.

To put the principle of mind renewal into practice, here is a general principle to follow to ensure you are eating the right amount for your body and not consistently overeating. It is called the SANE eating principle.

SANE stands for

- **S**tart when you are hungry
- **A**ppreciate every bite
- **N**o food is forbidden
- **E**nd when signaled.

Let's start with the *S*, which is paying attention to your body's hunger signals as the cue to eat. Many of us eat for reasons other than hunger. For example, you might eat simply because someone brought doughnuts in and left them out open the counter. You don't stop to consider whether you really need this food, but simply grab and devour a doughnut out of habit.

But this principle reminds you to be mindful of what you are eating and how much. In the case of the doughnut, you might still decide to have one due to hunger, but if not, you'll save it for later when you are. Chances are you will even enjoy it a lot more when you are hungry.

The next principle, '*A*ppreciate every bite', encourages you to slow down and enjoy your food. The brain has a built in appetite regulator that kicks in 20 minutes after you start eating. So if you are eating your meals in less time than that, it is possible that you are eating 2 or 3 times the amount that your body needs. When you eat more fruits and vegetables, you will automatically find yourself slowing down because these foods require more effort to chew and digest.

The third principle, *N*o food is forbidden, means that you don't forbid yourself to have any food just because society tells you that you shouldn't have it. Instead you examine the foods you eat and determine by personal choice which ones you will eat and which you will limit, if any. There is a big difference in limiting a food by personal choice versus only because "I can't have it because they told me not too." In the second scenario, you possibly set up a situation in which you want to rebel. However in the first one, there is no temptation to rebel, since it was your own personal eating decision.

The Mindful Eating Challenge, continued

Member Guide pg. 42

Pay attention to all the foods you eat and be sure that you select the ones that bring the most benefit to your body, both in taste and in function.

Finally, *E*nd when signaled is a reminder to stop eating when your body is satisfied. This will be just short of the fullness point. When you reach the satisfaction point, it's almost as if your body sighs, and your brain says, "Enough". Eating beyond this only stretches your stomach (nearly guaranteeing you'll eat more next time), and also giving your body extra calories it cannot use. When that happens, you will always end up carrying them around with you!

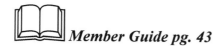 *Member Guide pg. 43*

Week 3 Homework Instructions

Leader Note: Explain the activities for homework to be completed <u>before</u> Week 4's class

Read Numbers 13 – 14:1-24

1. What instructions did God give to Moses?

   _____

   _____

2. What did the spies discover in the Valley of Eschol?

   _____

   _____

3. What report did most of the spies give when they returned to the congregation?

   _____

4. What did Joshua and Caleb say?

   _____

   _____

5. How did God respond to the spies and to Joshua and Caleb? Why do you think God responded this way?

   _____

   _____

Walk it Out Activities:

- Memorize next week's focus scripture.
- Copy the scriptures under the "God's Truth" column in the Limiting Beliefs table on index cards and meditate on them several times a day so they will renew your mind.
- **Mindful Eating Challenge:** Read the 'Mindful Eating' section. This week focus on practicing the SANE eating principle in how you eat. Continue tracking your food and water intake in your journal.

Week 4: I: Invest in Slimming Foods that Satisfy, Part 1

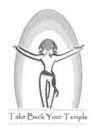

Take Back Your Temple

Week 4 Focus Scripture:

Along the bank of the river, on this side and that, will grow all kinds of trees used for food; their leaves will not wither, and their fruit will not fail. They will bear fruit every month, because their water flows from the sanctuary. Their fruit will be for food, and their leaves for medicine."

- Ezekiel 47:12 (NKJV)

Lesson Goals   In this lesson, you will learn how to:

Member Guide pg. 45

- Live out the ideal lifestyle for maximum health
- Determine the best foods to eat to lose weight
- Recognize portion sizes for healthy foods
- Fix your plate so that you can lose weight every time

Lesson Agenda

Quick Overview

- Welcome
- *Tense, Breathe, Jello Shake* exercise
- Recite this week's focus scripture
- Review the previous week's homework
- Review this week's lesson
- Homework Assignment

Leader Lesson Agenda

- (5 minutes) *Open in prayer.*
- (5 minutes) *Tense, Breathe, Jello Shake exercise.*
- (5 minutes) *Welcome everyone to class and document attendance.*
- (10 minutes) *Ask each person to recite this week's focus scripture.*
- (20 minutes) *Review the previous week's homework – answers follow on the next page.*
- (10 minutes) *Journal review* – Ask each person to turn in their Healthy Habits journals for review.

Ask the class to divide themselves into groups of 2 or 3. While you are reviewing the journals, ask each group to discuss the following question: *"What challenges did you encounter practicing SANE eating? How did/will you handle them?"*

After you have checked the journals, return them to their owners.

- (50 minutes) *Review this week's lesson and discuss*
- (10 minutes) Homework Assignment instructions
- (5 minutes) *Close in prayer and ask students for specific prayer needs/requests.*

Week 3 Homework - Answers

Leader Note: Have homework group discussion, asking for feedback for each question.

Read Numbers 13 – 14:1-24

1. What instructions did God give to Moses?

   "Send men to spy out the land of Canaan, which I am giving to the children of Israel; from each tribe of their fathers you shall send a man, every one a leader among them."

2. What did the spies discover in the Valley of Eschol?

   Then they came to the Valley of Eshcol, and there cut down a branch with one cluster of grapes; they carried it between two of them on a pole. They also brought some of the pomegranates and figs.

3. What report did most of the spies give when they returned to the congregation?

   "We are not able to go up against the people, for they are stronger than we." And they gave the children of Israel a bad report of the land which they had spied out, saying, "The land through which we have gone as spies is a land that devours its inhabitants, and all the people whom we saw in it are men of great stature. There we saw the giants (the descendants of Anak came from the giants); and we were like grasshoppers in our own sight, and so we were in their sight."

4. What did Joshua and Caleb say?

   "The land we passed through to spy out is an exceedingly good land. If the LORD delights in us, then He will bring us into this land and give it to us, 'a land which flows with milk and honey.' Only do not rebel against the LORD, nor fear the people of the land, for they are our bread; their protection has departed from them, and the LORD is with us. Do not fear them."

5. How did God respond to the spies and to Joshua and Caleb? Why do you think God responded this way?

   To the spies: They would not be allowed to see the Promised Land; Joshua and Caleb would be allowed to enter the land with an inheritance given for their descendants.

   - *Ask 1-2 students to contribute to this discussion.*

Our modern eating habits and lack of physical activity makes us sick, dulls our thinking, and robs us of the energy needed to fulfill our God-given purpose. That is a strong statement, but it is true. We are bombarded with stress, foods with poor nutritional value, and conveniences that make inactivity easy.

Our ancestors mostly ate foods that came from the ground or from the tree. These nutrient-rich, unprocessed foods have the power to heal, energize, and nourish our bodies. In addition to eating simple foods, they were physically active most days of the week.

To restore health, we need to return to our ancestors' simpler ways. It's helpful to think of health as like a fence:

The Weight Loss Fence™

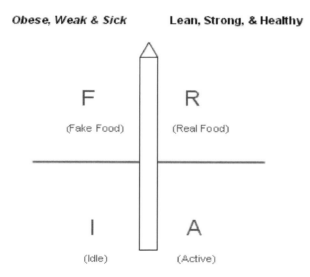

Every day, you make decisions about the food you eat and the physical activity you will do, which places you on the left side or right side of the fence. The right side choices help you lose weight if you need to, keep your body strong and supple, increase your energy and help you age gracefully, but less rapidly!

In contrast, the choices on the left side of the fence will cause weight gain (especially as you age and your rate of fat burning decreases), make your body weak and stiff, drain your energy, and make you age faster.

In this lesson, you will learn how to make "right side" choices in the foods you eat some that you can reach your weight loss goals faster. **Resolve to care more about what you put *in* your body than what you put *on* your body.**

Daniel's Example – Benefits of Vegetables and Water

Member Guide pg. 47

The bible gives you a great example of the impact of a healthy diet on the human body, that of Daniel in Daniel 1:8-16. Daniel and his friends were captives of the Babylonians, and Daniel decided that he was only going to eat the foods that God approved for his people to eat. So he asked the chief official for permission not to eat the king's rich food. After the official's hesitance, Daniel proposed a test: "For the next ten days, let us have only vegetables and water at mealtime. When the ten days are up, compare how we look with the other young men, and then decide what to do with us."

After those 10 days expired, Daniel and his friends looked healthier and better than the young men who ate the rich food. So that is the diet on which Daniel and his friends stayed - a great example to the king's men and to us today.

While you don't have to limit yourself to vegetables and water to be healthy, you can take advantage of their benefits by letting fiber-rich fruits and vegetables compose at least half of your diet. It was God's first food he directed man to eat and it is still the best for our bodies.

Leader Note: Ask for a volunteer to read Daniel's story from bible from Daniel 1:8-16.

Because fruits and vegetables are packed with fiber and water, which makes you feel full, it is hard to overeat them. You will feel full long before you consume enough calories to put you over your caloric limit for the day. On the other hand, it is very easy to overeat foods that are high in sugar and fat. Even in small amounts, they pack a lot of calories (measurement of energy that a food supplies to your body); so while you might not eat a lot in volume, you can exceed your calorie limit. Your ability to keep calories in line will ultimately make or break your weight loss efforts.

To prove the point, check out the typical regular size fast food lunch, usually around 1300 calories and compare it to the number of apples you would have to eat to take in that number of calories. You would have to eat about 20 apples in one sitting! Which do you think would ultimately leave you feeling fuller? Plus the apples will give you disease-fighting, age-proofing nutrients that are very scarce with the fast food meal.

Leader Note: Point out the comparison of the fast food lunch vs. the apples in the illustration.

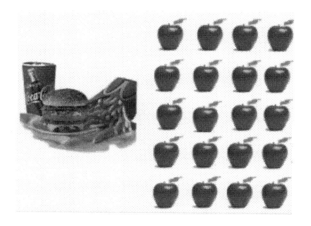

Another food group that will help you reach your best weight are *whole grain* products. Examples of these foods include whole grain bread, whole grain pastas, and brown rice. These products still have the bran in them, which is the grain's outer layer. Bran contains fiber, which makes you feel full and contributes to healthy digestion. It also contains disease-fighting vitamins and minerals - like iron, zinc, copper, magnesium, and B vitamins.

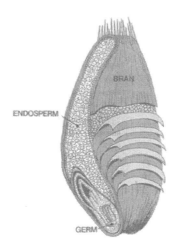

Unfortunately, many of the grain products we eat today are made with "white" grain, like white rice, pastas, and white bread. A "white" grain has had the bran stripped away from the grain, leaving only the white starchy center, the endosperm. Many are also put through a bleaching process.

Without the bran to slow down digestion, the grain breaks down very quickly into glucose (sugar) and causes a blood sugar spike. To handle this, your body releases insulin which is a hormone that moves sugar into the cells to restore your blood sugar balance. But sometimes the body does its job too well and releases an overload of insulin. Here is what happens next:

1. Your blood sugar lowers and your body strives to bring it back into balance quickly. You will crave food - and lots of it.

2. You will crave foods that are high in sugar or other white flour/rice products to bring your blood sugar up. Your body sees this as a necessary measure since it thinks that it's having a crisis.

3. The insulin that your body produced to handle the initial sugar rush is also a hormone that encourages fat storage. So those extra calories you consumed are very likely to be stored as fat.

The wisest thing is to choose whole grain products. On the ingredients list, look for the word *whole* in the grain description. If it doesn't have the word whole, it is not a whole grain even if it is brown in color!

Benefits of Healthy Fats

Member Guide pg. 49

A recent *Prevention Magazine* article outlined how the lack of Omega 3 fats in your diet can make you gain weight and may be behind some diseases like heart disease, diabetes, arthritis and cancer. Omega 3 fats are also essential to keeping your brain healthy, especially as you age.

The author said that Omega 3 fats start out in the green leaves of plants, which is the part of the plant with the highest metabolism. The green leaves are responsible for converting sunlight into sugars. Fish also have a lot of Omega 3 fatty acids because they eat seaweed and other green ocean plants.

In contrast, our modern diets are filled with another type of fat - Omega 6 fats. Instead of active fats, Omega 6s are storage fats. While Omega 3 fats are light and fluid, Omega 6 fats are thick or hard. Think about the difference between Olive oil and shortening. They can cause excessive blood clotting and make your arteries stiff.

Many processed foods are loaded with Omega 6 fats because food processors discovered that these fats increase the shelf life of products like cakes, cookies, chips, cereals, breads, and spreads – increasing their profits. In addition, cows and other animals are generally fed corn and soybeans (high in Omega 6 fats) to fatten them up for market, whereas in our grandparent's day, cows ate green grass. So their meat contains more Omega 6 fats.

While both Omega 6 fats and Omega 3 fats play a role in your body's health, the two compete for space in your cell membranes. So you want to eat more of the lighter, fluid Omega 3s.

So to gain maximum benefit from Omega 3s, eat more of these foods:

- Leafy green vegetables and other vegetables
- V8 and other mixed vegetable juices
- Beans
- Walnuts (watch the portions because they are high in calories
- Fish
- Foods prepared with olive oil, canola oil or flaxseed oil

To lighten up on the thicker Omega 6s, eat less of these foods:

- Fast food (loaded with Omega 6 fats)
- Prepared foods made with butter, margarine, cottonseed, soy, safflower, or sunflower oil
- Foods containing "hydrogenated" or "partially hydrogenated oils"

While you can supplement with fish oil or flax oil pills, they aren't as effective as eating the right foods. So for maximum health, make Omega 3 rich foods your best friend and limit your relationships with processed foods.

Eating Slimming Foods that Satisfy

Leader Note: *Ask for volunteers to read the chart of the food categories and their importance in weight loss aloud, one category per person - from **Page 50** in the Member Guide.*

The slimming foods are those that are mostly plant-based with a high fiber and/or water content, with moderate amounts of grains/starchy vegetables and lean meats/beans. Here is a table explaining why these foods are important in weight loss:

Food category	Importance in weight loss
Fruits and Vegetables	• Supply the body with 'B' vitamins, which help the body convert food into energy. • Can also supply 'C' vitamins, which help the body convert sugar into energy in the cells. • Contains fiber, which fills you up on fewer calories.
Lean Protein	• Helps support muscle growth and repair. Muscles help you burn extra fat even while you are resting. • Eating lean protein can also reduce your appetite, which can lower your caloric intake overall.
Whole grains/starchy vegetables	• Great source of fiber, which helps you feel full and satisfied on less calories • Aids digestion and helps prevent constipation
Water	• Drinking adequate water ensures that you aren't eating food when you are really thirsty. It's easy to get confused because the same part of the brain controls hunger and thirst. • It also ensures that the liver is supporting your fat burning process. Your liver is a backup organ for the kidneys, and the kidneys must have water to do their job. If they don't get it, the liver must assist - which means it has less time to help with fat burning. Give the kidneys plenty of water to do their job, so the liver can concentrate on doing its task.
Healthy fats	• Helps to slow the release of insulin into your blood stream which decreases your body's ability to store fat, particular belly fat • Slows down digestion which increases food satisfaction level

The Ideal Weight Loss Plate

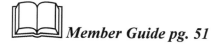 *Member Guide pg. 51*

As you can guess from the previous information, making most of your diet plant-based foods, like vegetables and fruits - along with water as your primary beverage - is the simplest and fastest way to lose weight every day and keep it off.

This is what your ideal daily pattern will look like approximately:

- Fruits and vegetables: 50%
- Grains and starchy vegetables: 25%
- Lean protein (meats and beans): 25%

And this is what your lunch and dinner plate will look like when prepared for maximum weight loss:

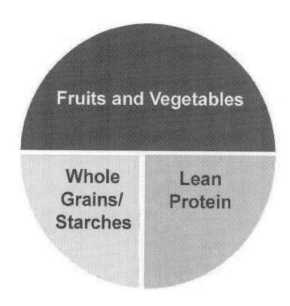

Breakfast will be slightly different. It's recommended that your plate be divided into thirds because it will be split evenly between your lean protein choice, a fruit portion, and a whole grain portion.

Practical Portion Sizes

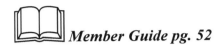 *Member Guide pg. 52*

Now that you know the best way to fix your plate, ensure that you are eating the right portion sizes with the foods on the plate. Even though you might fix your plate correctly, <u>piling it high with even the right foods will sabotage your goal</u>! Moderation is key.

In the right amounts, the slimming foods will make you feel satisfied without an excess of calories. The foods in **bold** are the best choices in each category since they are either high in fiber and/or vitamins and minerals that support your weight loss efforts.

	Note: The food portion advice given here is for women only. Men would require one extra portion of vegetables, fruit, starches, and healthy fats, plus two extra portions of lean protein.

	Tip: If you are not a big vegetable eater right now, place a checkmark besides the ones you know you like in this guide. Place a dash besides the ones you are willing to try. Each week, add 1 or 2 vegetable portions to your normal intake each day until you reach the recommended goal. There is an optional 'Health Tracking Log' in the Appendix that you can use to track your portion sizes.

*Leader Note: Review the portion size information and demonstrate with your hand how to determine portion sizes as indicated in the Members Guide from **Page 52-54**. Ask students to follow along with their hands so they can see how to gauge portion size.*

Vegetables: 5 portions per day (Strive to make half of these green leafy vegetables)

Green leafy vegetables – 1 cup per portion (size of 1 fist)

- **Brussels Sprouts**
- **Cabbage**
- **Collard Greens**
- Lettuce
- **Kale**
- **Mustard Greens**
- **Spinach**
- **Swiss Chard**
- **Turnips**
- Watercress

Note: Did you know that it is said that if you eat 2 ½ cups of vegetables each day, you can **prevent** most lifestyle-related diseases? Green leafy vegetables are rich in Alpha Lineolic Acid, an Omega 3 Fatty acid. This nutrient has been founds to help improve your ability to burn fat, make your joints more supple, makes your heart healthier and circulation flow more smoothly. Eating more vegetables and especially green leafy vegetables should help you reach your weight loss goals faster.

Other fibrous vegetables - 1/2 cup per portion (size of 1 cupped hand); 100% vegetable juice included.

- **Artichokes**
- **Asparagus**
- Avocado (also a healthy fat)
- Beets
- **Broccoli**
- **Carrots**
- **Cauliflower**
- Celery
- Chili Peppers
- **Cucumbers**
- Eggplant
- Garlic
- Gingerroot
- **Green beans**
- Leeks
- Mushrooms
- Okra
- Onions
- Parsley
- **Peppers**
- Radishes
- Scallions
- Sprouts
- **Squashes**
- **Tomatoes**
- Winter Squash
- **Zucchini**

Fruits: 2 portions per day

1 portion = 1 fist (medium piece of whole fruit) or ½ cup of fruit cocktail/salad or fruit juice per portion

- **Apples**
- Apricots
- Bananas
- **Blackberries**
- **Blueberries**
- Cantaloupes
- Cherries
- Cranberries
- **Figs**
- Grapefruit
- Grapes
- Honeydew Melon
- Kiwi Fruit
- Lemons
- Limes
- Mangoes
- Nectarines
- **Oranges**
- Papayas
- **Peaches**
- **Pears**
- Pineapples
- **Plums**
- **Prunes**
- Raisins
- **Raspberries**
- **Strawberries**
- Tangerines
- Tangelos
- Watermelon

Lean Protein: 3 portions per day

1 portion = Your palm (3 oz of meat, poultry or fish) or 1 cupped hand (1/2 cup beans or peas), 1 egg, 1 oz cheese, 1 cup yogurt

- Beef
- **Black Beans**
- **Black-eyed Peas**
- **Chicken**
- Cheese
- Eggs
- **Fish**
- **Garbanzo Beans**
- **Kidney Beans**
- **Lentils**
- **Lima Beans**
- Meat substitutes
- Milk
- **Pinto Beans**
- Split Peas
- **Turkey**
- Yogurt

Whole Grains or Starchy Vegetables: 3 portions per day

1 portion = 1 oz bread or cupped hand (1/2 cup pasta, corn, or small potato)

- Barley
- Bran/Whole Wheat Cereal (minimum 5 grams of fiber per portion)
- Bread (whole grain bread, bagel, waffle)
- **Brown Rice**
- Corn
- **Oats**
- **Pasta (whole grain)**
- **Popcorn (air popped)**
- **Sweet Potatoes/Yams**
- Tortillas (whole grain)

Plant-based Fats – 1 Portion a Day (Careful - High in Calories)

Nuts/seeds – ¼ cup approximately (1/2 cupped hand – palm only)

- **Almonds**
- Chocolate Chips (Bittersweet)
- **Flax seeds**
- **Macadamia nuts**
- Peanuts
- **Pistachios**
- **Sesame seeds**
- **Sunflower seeds**
- **Walnuts**

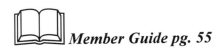

Week 4 Homework Instructions

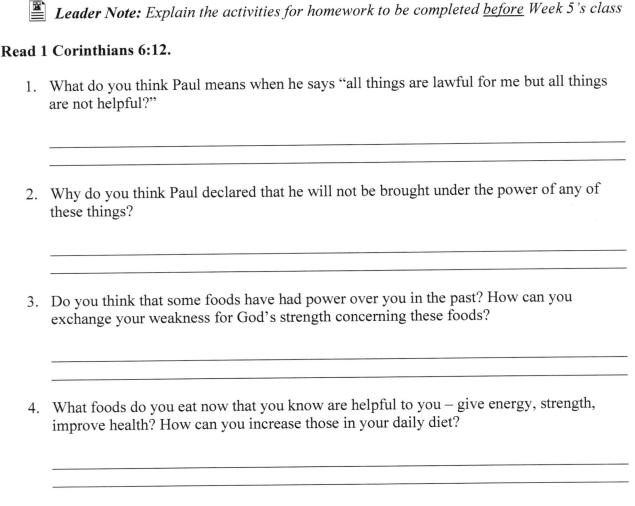 ***Leader Note:*** *Explain the activities for homework to be completed <u>before</u> Week 5's class*

Read 1 Corinthians 6:12.

1. What do you think Paul means when he says "all things are lawful for me but all things are not helpful?"

   _____

   _____

2. Why do you think Paul declared that he will not be brought under the power of any of these things?

   _____

   _____

3. Do you think that some foods have had power over you in the past? How can you exchange your weakness for God's strength concerning these foods?

   _____

   _____

4. What foods do you eat now that you know are helpful to you – give energy, strength, improve health? How can you increase those in your daily diet?

   _____

   _____

Walk it Out Activities:

- Memorize next week's focus scripture.
- In your daily eating this week, strive to fix your plate according to the "Ideal Weight Loss Plate".
- Review the portion sizes for the various food groups. When you fix your plate, also pay attention to ensure that you are eating reasonable portion sizes. Continue to write down your food intake in your journal.

Week 5: I: Invest in Slimming Foods that Satisfy, Part 2

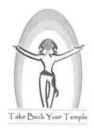

Take Back Your Temple

Week 5 Focus Scripture:

When you sit down to eat with a ruler,
Consider carefully what is before you;
And put a knife to your throat
If you are a man given to appetite.
Do not desire his delicacies,
For they are deceptive food.

- Proverbs 23:1-3 (NKJV)

Lesson Goals

Member Guide pg. 57

In this lesson, you will learn how to:

- Eat other favorite foods in balance
- Make wise choices when dining out
- Read food labels to make healthier choices
- Make preparing healthy meals easier

Lesson Agenda

Quick Overview

- Welcome
- *Tense, Breathe, Jello Shake* exercise
- Recite this week's focus scripture
- Review the previous week's homework
- Review this week's lesson
- Homework Assignment

Leader Lesson Agenda

- (5 minutes) *Open in prayer.*
- (5 minutes) *Tense, Breathe, Jello Shake exercise.*
- (5 minutes) *Welcome everyone to class and document attendance.*
- (10 minutes) *Ask each person to recite this week's focus scripture.*
- (20 minutes) *Review the previous week's homework – answers follow on the next page.*
- (10 minutes) *Journal review –* Ask each person to turn in their Healthy Habits journals for review.

Ask the class to divide themselves into groups of 2 or 3. While you are reviewing the journals, ask each group to discuss the following question: *"What progress did you make in fixing your plate according to the Ideal Weight Plate?"*

After you have checked the journals, return them to their owners.

- (50 minutes) *Review this week's lesson and discuss*
- (10 minutes) Homework Assignment instructions
- (5 minutes) *Close in prayer and ask students for specific prayer needs/requests.*

Week 4 Homework - Answers

Leader Note: *Have homework group discussion, asking for feedback for each question.*

Read 1 Corinthians 6:12.

1. What do you think Paul means when he says "all things are lawful for me but all things are not helpful?"

    - *Ask 1-2 students to contribute to this discussion.*

2. Why do you think Paul declared that he will not be brought under the power of any of these things?

    - *Ask 1-2 students to contribute to this discussion.*

3. Do you think that you have given some foods power over you in the past? How can you exchange your weakness for God's strength concerning these foods?

    - *Ask 1-2 students to contribute to this discussion.*

4. What foods do you eat now that you know are helpful to you – give energy, strength, improve health? How can you increase those in your daily diet?

    - *Ask 1-2 students to contribute to this discussion.*

In the previous week's lesson, you learned about the benefits of those foods closest to nature that help you lose weight if you need to, keep your body strong and supple, increase your energy and help you age gracefully.

However, everyone has less than healthy foods among their favorites and it is important to know how to eat these in balance so that you still enjoy the flavor of these foods, but avoid the consequences of overindulging in them.

Food is meant to be enjoyed, but so is your life as a whole. The pleasure of a meal lasts only a few minutes, yet the effects of that meal may stay with you for hours, or remain for days, weeks or even years if that food is not beneficial to your unique genetics.

As Proverbs 23:1 advises, consider carefully the food that is before you.

It is essential to pay close attention to how certain foods make you feel. Food is designed to heal, energize, and nourish you. If you are eating a food that makes you feel bloated, sick, tired, foggy, lazy, sluggish, sleepy, confused or irritable, then your body is giving you a loud and clear message that it doesn't like that food, even though your tongue may like the taste.

During the period when you are under the influence of that food, these ill feelings will certainly impact your ability to enjoy life to the fullest. If the negative pattern of lethargy, slothfulness, and lack of energy continues every day, it will ultimately impact your ability to fulfill your God-given purpose.

The focus scripture gives clear advice about self control when eating. In this case, *you* are the ruler since you are the one who chooses what and how much to feed your body. If a food tastes good while you are eating it, but it makes your body feel bad afterward, then to you it is a deceptive food.

Try cutting back on the portion size and see if your symptoms improve. If they do, then you may choose to limit that food or eliminate it. If you are experiencing these symptoms regularly, then investigate which foods are the worst culprits.

By writing things down in your journal, you can clearly see patterns and confront choices that you might ignore otherwise. You don't want any secrets between you and your body. This process will help you learn to trust your body to tell you what it needs and how it responds to certain foods. You can then use the information to make better choices overall and maintain your weight loss more easily.

Eating with Balance

Member Guide pg. 59

If you aim to eat healthy 90% of the time, then you can have whatever you want the other 10% - as long as you eat reasonable portion sizes. That's right…you can still have that scoop of mint chocolate chip ice cream, that piece of birthday cake, or macaroni and cheese…and still lose weight. So don't deprive yourself. You will actually end up hurting your weight loss efforts if you do, since deprivation is a classic set up for binge eating later.

Again, the important thing is to be sure you are eating reasonable portion sizes when you eat your favorite foods. Take the *thinnest* slice of cake or limit your ice cream and macaroni and cheese to ½ cup. While the amounts are small, they still pack a lot of calories compared to those in fruits and vegetables. That is why it is so easy to gain weight on a regular diet of these foods. Your goal is to get the flavor of your favorite foods without the excess.

When it comes to weight loss, it's not indulging occasionally in rich foods that trip you up; it is eating those foods on a daily basis. The calories add up quickly and translate to stored fat on your body!

So if managing your weight has been a challenge for you, the kindest thing for you to do now is to ensure that your daily eating habits are healthy ones. Then you'll have breathing room to enjoy those special occasions like birthdays, holidays, and other celebrations.

When those occasions occur, it is recommend using either of these two guidelines:

1. If you're eating a higher calorie food, then eat *half* of the amount you normally eat -OR-
2. Trade in the higher calorie food for a lighter alternative

Your ideal goal is to create a win/win situation for your body. You want to eat foods that you enjoy but also foods that are good for your body and help you maintain your energy, strength, vitality, and a pleasing shape. Doing this will help ensure that you are hitting the mark when it comes to your health and on the right path to taking back your temple.

Dining Out Tips

Member Guide pg. 60

Leader Note:
Review the Dining Out tips in this section and ask students for their tips.

Principle of the Half-size

One way you can help ensure that you eat the proper portions when dining out is to ask for a 'To Go' box right up front after placing your order. Many restaurants' portion sizes are huge – often 2 or 3 sizes larger than a normal serving! Asking for a box up front will help you avoid eating to excess.

Here is how: When your meal arrives with your 'To Go' box, immediately place half of your meal in it and set aside. You will really be getting two meals for the price of one. Also, you get to enjoy it twice!

This especially helps you if you are a member of the unofficial 'Clean Plate' club. A member of this club feels compelled to finish everything on his/her plate, which is usually a holdover from your parents' training during childhood. Putting half of your meal aside still allows you to finish everything on your plate, but you won't be consuming it all at once, which is overeating.

Other Dining Out Tips

- Split an entrée with a friend. You can always opt for an extra plate so you can share.
- Go lightly on the salad dressings because they can contain up to 400 calories just for ½ cup! So ask for the dressing on the side, then dip your fork into the dressing and stab into your salad. You'll still get the good taste, but without the extra calories.
- Also, favor the vinaigrette style dressings like Italian, Raspberry or Balsamic vinaigrette rather than the creamy ones like ranch and bleu cheese.
- Seek out dishes that are described as grilled, tomato-based, cooked in broth, au jus (or in its own juice). Also look for vegetable-rich dishes (of the non-starchy variety).
- Avoid or limit dishes described as rich, creamy, fried, or crispy.

Fast Food Tips

Member Guide pg. 61

Principle of the Small Size

With fast food, here is a major principle: **never** supersize your fast food meal. Even if it seems like a good deal money wise in the moment, it won't be ultimately from what it will cost you in terms of your future health and body satisfaction. Remember the phrase, "Supersize my meal, super size myself!"

Portion sizes have gotten out of control with fast food. Compare the size of a common cheeseburger 20 years ago versus today from the 'Portion Distortion Quiz' at the National Heart Lung and Blood Institute:

Leader Note: Point out the comparison photo of a cheeseburger 20 years ago to one today in the illustration.

   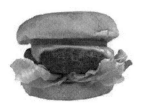

Cheeseburger 20 years Ago   **Cheeseburger Today**

333 calories   **590 calories**

You can see how eating out can escalate your odds of consuming too much food if you are not careful. So if you eat a fast food meal, order the smallest size that you possibly can. You might even order kids meals: you get what should actually be considered a normal adult portion size, plus you get a free prize. Money and health wise – it's a great deal!

Leader Note: Review the fast food tips and ask students to share any tips they have.

Other Fast Food Tips

- Make the fast food company's website your best friend – review it and decide what you will order before you go. Place your order at the drive through window. Put the food in the back seat because you will be surprised how much you can eat unconsciously while driving!
- Order your sandwich with whole grain bread if available.
- Order your sandwiches with only ketchup and mustard. Or if you like, order it plain and add low fat mayonnaise later.
- For sides, focus on tomato-based soups, corn on the cob, baked potato with chili, salad, or mixed vegetables rather than fried potatoes or onion rings.
- For beverages, choose water, small juice, or 1% milk.
- For pizza, order extra vegetables instead of extra meat; ask for light cheese and extra tomato sauce. When you get your slice, use a paper towel to blot some of the grease.
- Avoid the deep fried fish or chicken sandwiches. While chicken and fish are basically healthy, they aren't when deep fried in grease.
- Avoid sandwiches with multiple buns or meat patties

Eating at Home Tips

Member Guide pg. 62

Remember that the main idea with your eating plan is to make fruits and vegetables become 50% of more of your daily diet. Here are some quick tips on how to do that:

- Add vegetables to scrambled eggs or omelets like spinach, onions and mushrooms. You can also use a ¼ cup of salsa as a condiment with your omelets to add extra flavor and a "kick".
- Add fruit to your cereal like strawberries bananas and peaches
- Bulk up your sandwiches by added plenty of lettuce, tomato, and onion. This will help fill you up with fewer calories.
- Add ½ cup cooked vegetables to tomato soup or broth-based soup
- Add extra vegetables like tomatoes, onions, and peppers to spaghetti sauce and chili

When it comes to food preparation, select healthier cooking options like grilling, baking, roasting, sautéing, stir fry, or steaming. You still get great flavor without the fat.

If you ever need to have a frozen food meal at home instead of cooking dinner, here are some quick tips to help you choose wisely:

- Seek out vegetable-rich meals with chicken, turkey, fish, or beans
- Limit frozen meals with white rice and white pasta
- Choose meals that are 400 calories or less
- Choose meals that are lower in fat and sodium. Ideally your frozen food meal will have less than 600 mg of sodium and less than 10 grams of fat.

In setting yourself up for weight loss success, you must be mindful of creating a healthy "safety zone" around yourself. People tend to do what pleases their senses. If you don't have healthy foods in your home and workplace, and aren't prepared when you visit people or restaurants, then you may well be at the mercy of whatever you see or smell.

Please see the Appendix at the back of this guide for even more tips for food preparation and eating at home.

Eating at Work Tips

Member Guide pg. 63

Quick Tips for Work

- At work, keep a water bottle or jug on your desk that you may sip throughout the day. Many times, we eat food when our body is really crying for fluids.

- Keep a few snacks with you so you aren't at the mercy of the vending machines. Apples, oranges, small packs of raisins, almonds, walnuts or low sodium tomato or vegetable soup are some examples of food you can keep with you for emergencies. Proper planning is good for your health and waistline.

- Pack a healthy lunch. That way, you aren't always exposing yourself to food temptations. You will also save money this way as well!

Principle of the Serving Size

It is easy to become deceived when you are eating processed foods. Since many of them are full of either sugar or fat, which pack a lot of calories in small amounts, you might be eating more calories than you realize.

For example, let's say that you eat a pint of ice cream because you see that 250 calories is displayed in bold on the label. However, on further examination, you will see that each pint contains *4 servings*. So instead of the 250 calories that you thought, you were really consuming 1,000 calories!

For a typical inactive woman, it takes about 1,800 calories to maintain her weight. Since the ice cream was 1,000 calories, then it doesn't take a genius to figure out that a steady diet of foods like these would cause major weight gain over time. To prevent these deceptions from happening with you, a brief lesson on how to read food labels follows on the next page.

Leader Note: *Review the guidelines on food label reading on the next three pages, which also are found on pages **64-66** in the Member Guide.*

Food Label Reading – Example Macaroni and Cheese Box

Nutrition Facts Serving Size 1 cup (228g) Servings Per Container 2	The **Serving Size** shows the amount for a reasonable serving of the product, 1 cup in this example. **Servings per Container** shows how many servings are in the entire package. To see how many calories you'd consume if you ate the whole package, multiply the *Servings per Container* number by the *Calories* number.
Amount Per Serving **Calories** 250 Calories from Fat 110	**Calories** show the number of calories per serving, in this case 250 calories. 400 calories or more per serving is considered high calorie. Also check out the **Calories from Fat**. 110 Calories out of 250 comes from fat in this item, or almost half. The closer the *Calories from Fat* number is to the *Calories* number, the more fat the item has. A lower *Calories from Fat* number is better.
% Daily Value* **Total Fat** 12g 18% Saturated Fat 3g 15% *Trans* Fat 3g **Cholesterol** 30mg 10% **Sodium** 470mg 20% **Total Carbohydrate** 31g 10%	That **Total Fat**, **Cholesterol,** and **Sodium** show the amounts of these nutrients in each serving. Look at the % Daily Values. 5% or less is low, 20% or more is high. For these nutrients, *lower* is better.
Dietary Fiber 0g 0% Sugars 5g **Protein** 5g Vitamin A 4% Vitamin C 2% Calcium 20% Iron 4%	The **Dietary Fiber, Vitamin/Mineral (shown in blue)** listings display the amount of these nutrients in each serving. Look at the % Daily Values. 5% or less is low, 20% or more is high. For these nutrients, *higher* is better.

* Percent Daily Values are based on a 2,000 calorie diet. Your Daily Values may be higher or lower depending on your calorie needs.

	Calories:	2,000	2,500
Total Fat	Less than	65g	80g
Sat Fat	Less than	20g	25g
Cholesterol	Less than	300mg	300mg
Sodium	Less than	2,400mg	2,400mg
Total Carbohydrate		300g	375g
Dietary Fiber		25g	30g

The amounts that experts recommend we eat for fat, cholesterol, sodium, carbohydrates, and fibers are shown here. Note that these numbers are based on a 2,000 or 2,500 calorie diet. If you are eating a fewer number of calories, then the amounts recommended for fat, carbohydrates and fiber will lower also.

Food Label Ingredients – Example Yogurt

INGREDIENTS: CULTURED GRADE A REDUCED FAT MILK, APPLES, HIGH FRUCTOSE CORN SYRUP, CINNAMON, NUTMEG, NATURAL FLAVORS, AND PECTIN. CONTAINS ACTIVE YOGURT AND L. ACIDOPHILUS CULTURES.

When you are reading food label ingredients, they are listed in order of weight, from the most to the least. In the above label, reduced fat milk is listed first, because this yogurt contains more weight in reduced fat milk than any of its other ingredients.

A good guideline to follow when reading labels is: the shorter the list of ingredients, the better. This usually means there are fewer unhealthy additives and preservatives. Also, if a product either contains an item that you don't know, or you can't pronounce, this is a good indicator not to put it into your body (like monosodium glutamate, for instance).

Here are some other things to keep in mind when reading labels:

Sugars

When you are reading labels, look for any hidden sugars in the product. You will be looking for lower sugar items, so you don't want sugar to be listed as one of the first 4 ingredients in the product.

However, sugar is not always listed as "sugar". Here are some of the other names for sugar you should learn:

Brown sugar	Glucose	Molasses
Corn sweetener	High-fructose corn syrup	Raw sugar
Corn syrup	Invert sugar	Sucrose
Dextrose	Lactose	Refined Sugar
Fructose	Maltose	Syrup
Fruit juice concentrates	Malt syrup	

Whole Grains

When you are looking for whole grain products, like breads and pastas, don't just read the manufacturer's hype on the front of the package or buy the product just because it is brown.

Often, a manufacturer might say "made with whole grain" on the front, but when you read the ingredients, you see that the grain is way down on the list. Also, manufacturers sometimes add molasses to bread to turn it brown, but the product itself is still not a whole grain.

You want to ensure that the whole grain products you buy have one of the following ingredients listed first on the label ingredients:

Brown rice	Whole oats
Bulgur	Whole rye
Graham flour	Whole wheat
Oatmeal	Wild rice
Whole grain corn	

Trans Fats

Eating trans fats increases your risk of developing heart disease. Trans fats are found in many processed foods like cookies and crackers because it makes them last longer on the store shelves.

When you are reading your food labels, beware of the ingredient 'fully or partially hydrogenated vegetable oil' on the list. If the product contains this ingredient, it has trans fat in it. I recommend replacing that item with another choice without the trans fat.

*Leader Note: Do the following Food Label reading activity if time permits – make copies of the label on the next page before class, pass out the copies, and ask students to use the information from **Page 64-66** in the Member Guide to answer the questions below the label.*

SAMPLE FOOD LABEL - READING QUIZ

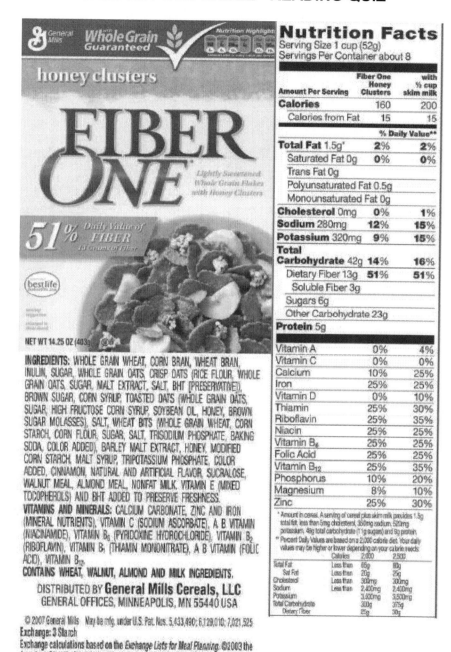

1. If you ate 2 cups of this cereal, how many calories would you consume? _____

2. Does this product contain whole grains? How do you know? _____

3. What sources of sugar do you see on this label? _____

Answers to the Food Label Reading Quiz:

1. 320 Calories

2. Yes; The whole grain ingredients have the word "whole" in them – such as whole grain wheat, whole grain oats, and bran (bran is the substance that makes a "whole grain" whole because the bran is the outer portion of the grain. In white bread and grain products the bran has been removed, so it is no longer whole).

3. Sugar, Brown Sugar, Corn Syrup, High Fructose Corn Syrup, Honey, Molasses, Barley Malt Extract, Sucrolose

Ideally, you don't want sugar to be listed in the first 4 ingredients – even though this item has many different sources of sugar, according to the label they are in smaller amounts. The largest percentage of ingredients this product contains are whole grain items.

Week 5 Homework Instructions

Leader Note: *Explain the activities for homework to be completed <u>before</u> Week 6's class*

Read Proverbs 21:5.

1. According to the scripture, what do the plans of the diligent lead to?

   _____

   _____

2. According to the scripture, what happens to those who are hasty?

   _____

   _____

3. Regarding your health habits in the past (eating and physical activity), would say that you've planned diligently, hastily, or not planned at all? If you've either planned hastily or never made plans, what can you do differently now to achieve success?

   _____

   _____

Read Proverbs 23:1-3.

1. The scripture advises to exercise discipline when you eat with a "ruler" because of deceptive foods. What deceptive foods do you eat regularly that make you feel sluggish, bloated or otherwise unwell physically? What can you do to limit these foods in your diet to make room for ones that improve your health?

   _____

   _____

   _____

Walk it Out Activities:

- Memorize next week's focus scripture.
- Review the tips under the Dining Out, Fast Food, Eating at Home, and At Work tips. Pick at least three of the tips that you will practice.
- In your daily eating this week implement the tips of your choice. Write down any benefits or challenges you experienced in your journal.

Week 6: S: Slim, Stretch, and Strengthen your Body

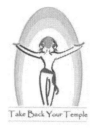

Take Back Your Temple

Week 6 Focus Scripture:

But I discipline my body and bring it into subjection, lest, when I have preached to others, I myself should become disqualified.

- 1 Corinthians 9:27 (NKJV)

Lesson Goals

Member Guide pg. 69

In this lesson, you will learn how to:

- Increase your fat-burning ability up to 9x with any activity
- Burn fat even at rest with strength training
- Improve your flexibility, balance, and body shape

Lesson Agenda

Quick Overview

- Welcome
- *Tense, Breathe, Jello Shake* exercise
- Recite this week's focus scripture
- Review the previous week's homework
- Review this week's lesson
- Homework Assignment

Leader Lesson Agenda

- (5 minutes) *Open in prayer.*
- (5 minutes) *Tense, Breathe, Jello Shake exercise.*
- (5 minutes) *Welcome everyone to class and document attendance.*
- (10 minutes) *Ask each person to recite this week's focus scripture.*
- (20 minutes) *Review the previous week's homework – answers follow on the next page.*
- (10 minutes) *Journal review* – Ask each person to give you their Healthy Habits journals for review; assure them that you aren't judging what is in it - only compliance with the assignment to provide accountability.

Ask the class to divide themselves into groups of 2 or 3. While you are reviewing the journals, ask each group to discuss the following question: *"Which eating tips did you practice from last week? What did you do well? What will you do differently next week?"*

After you have checked the journals, return them to their owners.

- (50 minutes) *Review this week's lesson and discuss*
- (10 minutes) Homework Assignment instructions
- (5 minutes) *Close in prayer and ask students for specific prayer needs/requests.*

Week 5 Homework - Answers

Read Proverbs 21:5.

1. According to the scripture, what do the plans of the diligent lead to?

   To plenty

2. According to the scripture, what happens to those who are hasty?

   To poverty

3. Regarding your health habits in the past (eating and physical activity), would say that you've planned diligently, hastily, or not planned at all? If you've either planned hastily or never made plans, what can you do differently now to achieve success?

   - *Ask 1-2 students to contribute to this discussion.*

Read Proverbs 23:1-3.

1. The scripture advises to exercise discipline when you eat with a "ruler" because of deceptive foods. What deceptive foods do you eat regularly that make you feel sluggish, bloated or otherwise unwell physically? What can you do to limit these foods in your diet to make room for ones that improve your health?

   - *Ask 1-2 students to contribute to this discussion.*

As you lose weight, you want to be sure that your body is reshaping itself into an appearance that pleases you. You want to regain that pep in your step - to meet any physical challenge, fulfill your life's purpose…and have energy to spare.

In this step, there are three areas in which you accomplish this goal:

- Slim: This type of exercise is aerobic, which helps your body burn fat efficiently. However, we are going to turbo-charge your exercise so that you'll get faster results in less time.

- Stretch: These exercises help decrease your risk of injury, increase your flexibility, regain your balance, and lengthen your muscles, giving you a leaner appearance. They are also great for re-establishing your spirit/mind/body connection, which is vital to keeping you on track.

- Strengthen: Strengthening exercises target your muscles, which add shape to the body. By working on your muscle tone, you will also increase your body's ability to burn fat.

  Muscles are calorie incinerators. Each pound of muscle burns 40 calories a day just to stay alive while a pound of fat burns only 3 calories. Increasing your lean muscle mass helps you lose fat even at rest so that it is easier to maintain your fat loss in the long run.

As you work your weight loss plan, you will need to keep track of your progress. You may be surprised to learn that the scale is not the best way to measure your results. Why? Because a typical scale does not show you how much of your body composition is muscle versus fat. If you gain muscle, the scale will show a weight gain, which most of us assume is a bad thing.

In this case, it is not. Muscle not only burns more calories than fat, but it also takes up less room than fat. So if your clothing size drops, but your weight stays the same or you gain scale weight don't panic. You are losing fat, but you gained muscle. And fat is what you want to get rid of so you are on the right track!

Now let's learn about the best exercises to stretch, slim, and strengthen your body.

,

Stretching Yourself Out

Stretching is an essential part of your weight loss plan because in addition to increasing your flexibility, it also provides a way for you to relax, de-stress, and improve your posture. An improved posture may help you appear slimmer, even before you lose a pound.

Member Guide pg. 71

Your stretching program will also renew the connection between your mind and body. It's very easy to lose touch with your body and its needs. But your stretching time is designed to be a time in which you relax, breathe deeply, and enjoy your body and all it does for you.

Finally, stretching may also enhance your weight loss program due to extra calories you can burn. Researchers have shown that adding extra movement into your day, whether through stretching or even simple fidgeting, can burn up to 350 calories per day!

Stretching is the most convenient exercise there is. After all, you don't need a special time or place to stretch. At home or at work, you can just stand up, push your arms toward the ceiling, and stretch. One of the best times to stretch your body is after you take a warm shower or bath. Take each of your joints through their fullest range of motion.

You can stretch every day, which is safe for most people to do. As you age, your muscles start to lose their elasticity and the tissues around your joints thicken. However, deliberately bending, moving, and stretching will help to keep joints flexible and muscles elastic.

Stretching daily will help make your other physical activities easier. Here are two points to keep in mind with your stretching program:

***Leader Note:** Review the bulleted stretching tips in this section.*

- Never stretch cold muscles. Warm up by walking in place, dancing, or other physical activity for 5 minutes.
- Start your stretching workout with deep breathing and continue throughout your session. Try to work up to 50 deep breaths per workout
- Stretch slowly and just to the point where you feel tightness. **Never** go to the point of pain. With practice and patience, your muscles will loosen up and you'll be able to stretch farther.
- Hold your stretch for about 30 seconds without bouncing.

The stretching exercises that follow are those that can be done anytime during the course of your day. Do them as often as you can throughout the day.

Neck, Back and Shoulder Stretch

The neck, back and shoulders are particularly vulnerable to tension and stress. This easy stretch will help to relax your muscles and is also useful to do after any activity that makes you feel stiff, like sitting at a desk for long periods or working at a computer.

Member Guide pg. 72

Leader Note:
Ask the class to stand up and follow along with you as you demonstrate the stretching exercises on **Page 72-73** *in the Member Guide.*

Step	Action
1	Stand with your feet shoulder-width apart, your knees straight but not locked, and your hands clasped in front of you.
2	Rotate your hands so that your palms are facing the ground; then raise your arms to about chest height.
3	Gently press your palms away from your body. You should feel a stretch in your neck and upper back and along your shoulders.
4	Hold the stretch for a slow count of 20 to 30, breathing throughout.
5	Release the stretch and repeat. **Note:** You can also do this exercise when sitting down periodically during the day.

Chest and Arm Stretch   This reaching stretch improves your flexibility in your arms, chest, and front of your shoulders.

Member Guide pg. 73

Step	Action
1	Stand with your arms at your sides and your feet about shoulder-width apart.
2	Extend both arms behind your back and clasp your hands together, if possible, pulling your shoulders back.
3	Raise your arms slightly, holding the stretch for a slow count of 20 to 30, breathing throughout.
4	Release the stretch and repeat.

Leg and Calf Stretch

This exercise helps you loosen the muscles in the back of the legs and calves. It's a great exercise to do while you are watching television.

Member Guide pg. 74

Leader Note:
Ask everyone to sit down and follow along with you as you demonstrate the leg and calf stretch exercise.

Step	Action
1	Sit forward in a chair with your knees bent and feet flat on the floor.
2	Extend your right leg in front of you, placing your right heel on the floor, and keeping your ankle relaxed. Don't lock your knee. Slowly lean forward at the hips, bending toward your right toes, keeping your back straight and your head lifted.
3	Hold the stretch for a slow count of 20 to 30, breathing throughout.
4	Sit up straight again and flex your right ankle so that your toes are pointing up toward the ceiling. Again, lean forward at the hips, bending toward your right toes and hold the stretch for a slow count of 20 to 30, breathing throughout.
5	Release the stretch and repeat with your left leg.

Blow Torch Your Fat

Member Guide pg. 75

Leader Note: Review the types of aerobic exercise in the bulleted list below and ask students to place a checkmark by the activities they can do.

Just think of the excess fat on your body as stored up energy that is waiting to be used.

How will you do it? When you add a technique called HIIT (High Intensity Interval Training) to a typical workout, you can burn up to 9 times more fat in the hours after the workout is complete. So even when you are watching television or working at your desk later on that day, your body will still be burning fat like crazy.

HIIT is performing a heart-healthy activity (like walking, running, biking, jump roping, swimming, or stair climbing) by alternating fast, high intensity moves with slower, lower intensity moves during each session. By adding these brief, challenging segments to your workout, your body is forced to raid its fat stores in the hours afterwards to get the energy it needs for your recovery.

Have you ever seen how lean Olympic sprinters look? Think of HIIT as adding Olympic sprints into your typical workout. The sprints only last about 30 seconds at a time, but you repeat them several times in your workout. The great thing about adding HIIT to your workouts is that you won't have to spend hours in the gym or on the treadmill to get results. You will be getting better results in less time and you'll help alleviate workout boredom.

For maximum benefit, it is recommended that you perform HIIT exercise at 2-3 times a week, allowing at least 24 hours between workouts. For example, you can HIIT on Monday, Wednesday, and Friday. Pick any of the following physical activities for your primary activity. You can also mix and match:

- Walking (outdoor or treadmill)
- Swimming
- Dancing
- Biking
- Skating
- Stair Climbing
- Elliptical Machine
- Rowing Machine
- Jump Roping

 If you have heart disease, high blood pressure, diabetes, joint problems like arthritis, or are older than age 60, then please consult your doctor before starting an exercise routine.

How to HIIT

Member Guide pg. 76

To start, you want to warm up for 5 minutes. You can just walk in place for 5 minutes and then take a couple of minutes to stretch. Your ultimate goal is to work up to 45 minutes, but if you are just starting to exercise, just set a goal to work out for 20 minutes. And if that is too much, then start with 10 minutes. You want to work with your body and pay attention to what it tells you.

Then, follow this pattern or a similar one throughout your workout:

- Go fast for 30 seconds
- Recover for 3 minutes at a moderate pace
- Go fast for 30 seconds
- Recover for 3 minutes at a moderate pace

…and so on

Finish your workout with a 5 minute cool down and stretch. During your 'Go fast' segments, you really want to challenge yourself. Go as fast as you can. Step out of your comfort zone and test your limits. Be sure to keep your body relaxed and breathe deeply. Also be sure that you've had plenty of water to drink before starting your workout. If at any time you start to feel nauseous, dizziness, or pain then slow down. If the discomfort continues, then stop. You want to challenge yourself, but you also want to use common sense.

During your recovery periods, go at a moderate pace so that it is still challenging, but comfortable.

If you haven't been exercising for a while, then just strive to go at a moderate pace without the HIIT segments your first 2 weeks. Then when you are ready, just add 1 or 2 challenge segments, paying attention to how your body responds. It will start to adapt to this new challenge and then you can add on as you feel comfortable. **Always** listen to your body. Some days your body might ask you to go easy and some days it might be ready for a greater challenge. Whatever energy it gives you to work with that day, use it!

For those who are reasonably healthy, then really go for it during those challenge segments. The more you do the more after burn you will create when the workout is over. Plus when your workout is over, you will be amazed at your feelings of accomplishment, well being, and energy. You will also be astonished by how quickly your body will change!

Reshape Your Body

Member Guide pg. 77

Leader Note: Ask students to look at the muscle vs. fat illustration (fat is on the top, the muscle on the bottom) and consider the difference.

Your muscles are the engine of your body. When you increase muscle, they will burn your excess fat—even while you sleep! Adding just 4 ½ pounds of muscle to your body burns as many calories as running one mile every day. And because muscles take up less room than fat, you can drop clothing sizes even if the scale isn't moving that much.

To illustrate the point, here is the difference in appearance and size between 5 pounds of muscle verses 5 pounds of fat.

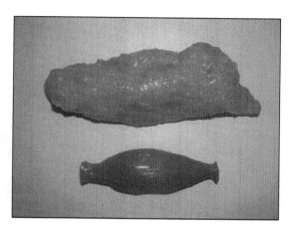

Five pounds of muscle on your body uses 200 calories a day just to stay alive. The same amount of fat only uses 15 calories. So think of muscles as the hardworking laborers of your body, while your fat cells are freeloaders!

After you reach age 35, you lose ½ pound of muscle each year and gain 1 ½ pounds of fat if you don't strength train. The half pound of muscle you lose means that you are burning 20 less calories each day. It doesn't sound like much, but that translates to gaining 10 pounds every 5 years! Regular strength training helps prevent this from occurring.

Many women are worried about looking too bulky and masculine if they strength train. However, the hormone testosterone is responsible for muscle building and women have very little of it. Female body builders use very heavy weight, strict diets, and some use performance enhancers to gain bulk. This program will strengthen and shape your muscles without the bulk.

You can strength train using your own body weight, using dumbbells, weight machines, or resistance bands. The following routine uses dumbbells.

 If you have heart disease, high blood pressure, diabetes, joint problems like arthritis, or are older than age 60, then please consult your doctor before starting a strength training routine.

Equipment you Need

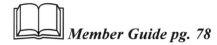 *Member Guide pg. 78*

To perform the recommended strength program, you will need three sets of dumbbell weights:

• Three pounds
• Five pounds
• Eight pounds

 Note: The recommended weight sizes are for women only. Men would need heavier weights to see strength gains.

You can get your weights at a discount store or sporting goods store.

According to the American College of Sports Medicine (ACSM), the goal with each strength training exercise is to complete eight to 12 repetitions (rep) of each exercise.

After you complete the recommended number of reps, rest for a minute or two, and then perform another set of the exercise. You may perform up to three sets of each exercise.

Keep the following tips in mind:

- Start with the heaviest weight you can use with good form. Ideally, it should be heavy enough so that the last 2 or 3 repetitions are challenging to do.
- If your muscles ever start to tremble when you are attempting to lift a weight, it is too heavy for you. Lighten up.
- When you can easily perform the recommended repetitions and sets using your current weight, move up to the next level weight.
- Use the following speed when lifting: 3 seconds to lift, 1 second to pause, 3 seconds to lower.
- Make your movements smooth, extending the muscle through its full range of motion. **Never** jerk the weights.
- Breathe deeply and evenly, inhale during the easy part of the movement, exhale when it is challenging.
- Perform your strength training workout 2 or 3 times a week on alternate days.

*Leader Note: Review the bulleted strength training guidelines above and then demonstrate the exercises on the following four pages (**Page 79-82** in the Member Guide.)*

Chair Stand

This exercise strengthens and shapes your hips, thighs, and backside. It will also make other exercises like walking, climbing stairs, or dancing easier.

Step	Action
1	In front of a sturdy, armless chair, stand with feet slightly more than shoulder-width apart. Extend your arms out so they are parallel to the ground and lean forward a little at the hips.
2	Making sure that your knees **never** come forward past your toes, lower yourself in a slow, controlled motion, to a count of four, until you reach a near-sitting position.
3	Pause. Then, to a count of two, slowly rise back up to a standing position. Keep your knees over your ankles and your back straight.
4	Repeat 10 times for one set. Rest for one to two minutes. Then complete a second set of 10 repetitions.

If the exercise is too hard, you can use your hands for assistance. Also, if you are unable to go all the way down, place a couple of pillows on the chair or only squat down four to six inches.

Overhead Press

You will tone up several muscles in your arms, upper back, and shoulders with this exercise. It will also help you wave bye-bye to back of the arm flab.

Step	Action
1	Stand or sit in an armless chair with feet shoulder-width apart. With a dumbbell in each hand, raise your hands, palms facing forward, until the dumbbells are level with your shoulders and parallel to the floor.
2	To a count of two, slowly push the dumbbells up over your head until your arms are fully extended—but don't lock your elbows. Be sure to keep your wrists straight.
3	Pause. Then, to a count of four, slowly lower the dumbbells back to shoulder level, bringing your elbows down close to your sides.
4	Repeat 10 times for one set. Rest for one to two minutes. Then complete a second set of 10 repetitions.

Calf Raise

This exercise gives you shapely calves and ankles and helps maintain your stability and balance as you age.

Step	Action
1	Stand with feet shoulder-width apart near a counter or sturdy chair. Hold on to the chair or counter for balance, but don't lean on it.
2	To a count of four, slowly push up as far as you can, onto the balls of your feet and hold for two to four seconds.
3	Then, to a count of four, slowly lower your heels back to the floor.
4	Repeat 10 times for one set. Rest for one to two minutes. Then complete a second set of 10 repetitions.

Biceps Curl with Rotation

This exercise tones the front of your arms and makes lifting objects like milk jugs easier.

Step	Action
1	With a dumbbell in each hand, stand or sit in an armless chair, with feet shoulder-width apart, arms at your sides, and palms facing your thighs.
2	To a count of two, slowly lift up the weights so that your forearms rotate and palms face in toward your shoulders, while keeping your upper arms and elbows close to your side—as if you had a newspaper tucked beneath your arm. Keep your wrists straight and dumbbells parallel to the floor.
3	Pause. Then, to a count of four, slowly lower the dumbbells back toward your thighs, rotating your forearms so that your arms are again at your sides, with palms facing your thighs.
4	Repeat 10 times for one set. Rest for one to two minutes. Then complete a second set of 10 repetitions.

Pelvic Tuck

This exercise tightens your stomach muscles and backside. It also improves your posture.

Step	Action
1	On the floor or on a firm mattress, lie flat on your back with your knees bent, feet flat, and arms at your sides, palms facing the ground.
2	To a count of two, slowly roll your pelvis so that your hips and lower back are off the floor, while your upper back and shoulders remain in place.
3	Pause. Then, to a count of four, slowly lower your pelvis all the way down.
4	Repeat 10 times for one set. Rest for a minute or two. Then complete a second set of 10 repetitions.

Back Extension

This exercise complements the pelvic tuck exercise by strengthening the muscles of the lower back. Many people suffer lower back pain because of an imbalance in strength between the stomach and back muscles. This exercise can help prevent this pain by restoring this balance.

Step	Action
1	Lie on the floor facedown, with two pillows under your hips. Extend your arms straight overhead on the floor.
2	To a count of two, slowly lift your right arm and left leg off the floor, keeping them at the same level.
3	Pause. Then, to a count of four, slowly lower your arm and leg back to the floor.
4	Repeat 10 times for one set, and then switch to left arm with right leg for another 10 repetitions.
5	Rest for a minute or two. Then complete a second set of 10 repetitions.

Week 6 Homework Instructions

📓 ***Leader Note:*** *Explain the activities for homework to be completed <u>before</u> Week 7's class*

Read 1 Corinthians 9:27 and answer the following question.

1. What reason did Paul give for disciplining his body?

   _____

   _____

2. What do you think it means to be "disqualified"?

   _____

   _____

Read 1 Corinthians 6:19-20 and answer the following question.

3. Paul states believers should glorify God in their body and spirit. How can you glorify God in this way?

   _____

   _____

Read James 1:2-8 and answer the following question.

4. James states that a double minded man is unstable in all his ways. Have you been double minded when it comes to exercise? If so, what can you do differently to regain stability in this area?

   _____

   _____

Walk it Out Activities:

- Memorize next week's focus scripture.
- Review the exercises regarding how to slim, stretch, and strengthen your body. Assess your current exercise habits and plan how you can slowly implement the recommendations.
- Write down your planned activities in your health journal and document your follow through.

Week 7: E: Expect Tests and Be Prepared

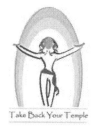

Take Back Your Temple

Week 7 Focus Scripture:

No temptation has overtaken you except such as is common to man; but God is faithful, who will not allow you to be tempted beyond what you are able, but with the temptation will also make the way of escape, that you may be able to bear it.

- 1 Corinthians 10:13 (NKJV)

Lesson Goals

Member Guide pg. 85

In this lesson, you will learn how to:

- Recognize common weight loss challenges
- Handle common weight loss challenges
- Create an action plan for the challenges that you may face

Lesson Agenda
Quick Overview

- Welcome
- *Tense, Breathe, Jello Shake* exercise
- Recite this week's focus scripture
- Review the previous week's homework
- Review this week's lesson
- Homework Assignment

Leader Lesson Agenda

- (5 minutes) *Open in prayer.*
- (5 minutes) *Tense, Breathe, Jello Shake exercise.*
- (5 minutes) *Welcome everyone to class and document attendance.*
- (10 minutes) *Ask each person to recite this week's focus scripture.*
- (20 minutes) *Review the previous week's homework – answers follow on the next page.*
- (10 minutes) *Journal review* – Ask each person to turn in their Healthy Habits journals for review.

Ask the class to divide themselves into groups of 2 or 3. While you are reviewing the journals, ask each group to discuss the following question: *"What physical activities did you practice this week? What is your plan for establishing this as a regular habit?"*

After you have checked the journals, return them to their owners.

- (50 minutes) *Review this week's lesson and discuss*
- (10 minutes) Homework Assignment instructions
- (5 minutes) *Close in prayer and ask students for specific prayer needs/requests.*

Week 6 Homework - Answers

Leader Note: *Have homework group discussion, asking for feedback for each question.*

Read 1 Corinthians 9:27 and answer the following question.

1. What reason did Paul give for disciplining his body?

   So that he would not be disqualified when he preached to others.

2. What do you think it means to be "disqualified"?

   - *Ask 1-2 students to contribute to this discussion.*

Read 1 Corinthians 6:19-20 and answer the following question.

4. Paul states believers should glorify God in their body and spirit. How can you glorify God in this way?

   - *Ask 1-2 students to contribute to this discussion.*

Read James 1:2-8 and answer the following question.

5. James states that a double minded man is unstable in all his ways. Have you been double minded when it comes to exercise? If so, what can you do differently to regain stability in this area?

   - *Ask 1-2 students to contribute to this discussion.*

Lesson
Introduction

Member Guide
pg. 86

Life happens. You might have the best intention of staying on track with your weight loss goals, but then someone brings donuts into the office.

That is a test.

Or your Great Aunt Gertrude insists that you eat all the enormous piece of red velvet cake she just placed in front of you.

That's a test.

Or it's night time and you aren't really hungry, but the kitchen seems to be calling you.

That's a test.

You get the picture. So an important part of the *Take Back Your Temple* process is to think about the situations that can pull you off track and come up with solutions in advance to deal with them before they damage your waistline.

A good way to start this step is to think about some of your previous efforts with losing weight. At what point did you give up? Were there any situations that discouraged you or made you say, "Forget it?" You've already paid for that experience, so you might as well take advantage of it by coming up with a plan to deal with the pitfalls if the issue comes up again.

So remember that one of God's promises is that the temptations you face come bundled with the solution for overcoming them. If you don't see it, then ask God to show you the solution. Temptations are permitted so that we might overcome them. You are more than a conqueror through Jesus Christ, so it is time to start taking back some territory!

This lesson will cover some common tests or temptations that you might face - along with some actions to handle them. You'll also have a worksheet to use to think about your own potential tests and your solutions to deal with them.

**Night-time
Eating**

***Member Guide
pg. 87***

***Leader Note:
Review the tips
in this section
and ask
students to
share their
tips.***

If you are tempted to eat late at night, the following tips can help. Make a copy of them and post them on your refrigerator. Try at least two of these strategies when you are tempted to eat:

- Listen to praise music to calm down and change the atmosphere
- Brush your teeth after dinner; swish your mouth with minty or intense cinnamon-flavored mouthwash
- Drink a cup of hot herbal tea with the herb Stevia for sweetness. You can find Stevia in your local health food store.
- Be aware that most fast food commercials air between 8-10 p.m.; you can either choose not to watch T.V. during those times or occupy yourself when the commercials come on.
- Do some simple stretching exercises to relax and unwind.
- Are you tired? Then don't use food as a means to stay up longer. Go to bed.
- Decide on three actions to take instead of eating, such as listening to music, playing with your child, or reading scripture.

Most importantly, **never** starve yourself; not eating enough during the day is a classic setup for overeating at night.

Office Junk Food

Member Guide pg. 87

You don't want to be blindsided by food temptations, so keep some high fiber snacks with you at all times - like apples, pears, orange, almonds, or an energy bar (less than 150 calories). This way, when temptations come, you will have something healthy to fall back on. And if you decide to indulge, then you will be more likely to keep your portion sizes reasonable since you won't feel very hungry.

Hungry at the Grocery Store

Leader Note: Review the tips in this section and ask students to share their tips.

You may have heard the tip to never shop hungry. But suppose you become hungry while you are shopping? When you're in the store, go ahead and purchase a high fiber fruit like an apple, a pear, or an orange. You might also purchase bottled water. When you're driving home, drink the water and eat the fruit, with the rest of the groceries safely in the trunk.

Snacks that are calorie dense, like trail mix, nuts, and dried fruit are not the best choice to eat while driving. These contain a lot of calories in even small amounts and you can eat more than you realize since your attention is divided with driving. It's best to satisfy your hunger with the fewest calories possible.

Bottomless Food Pits

Have you ever had the experience of sitting down to watch T.V. with a bag of buttered popcorn or potato chips in hand, and then found yourself reaching into an empty bag a short while later? If so, then you fell into a bottomless food pit. Below are some examples and how to deal with them:

Member Guide pg. 88

Leader Note:
Review the tips in this section and ask students to share their tips.

Ask students if there are any bottomless food pits that they have fallen into consistently and now that they know how to avoid them, what they will do differently.

Jumbo sized tubs/bags of popcorn: Even though you say you are going to share these with everyone else at the movies, somehow it winds up parked in your lap. Instead, buy everyone their own box and make sure yours is the smallest size available. Also, order the regular buttered popcorn, not the extra buttered kind. You will find that the regular style is buttery enough by itself.

Super-sized fast food meals: If you must go to a fast food restaurant, pass up the super size meals. Get the regular or junior sizes. You will still get the flavor without the extra calories. Remember the saying, "Super size your meal, super size yourself."

Whole takeout pizzas: Avoid parking the open box in front of you and eating directly from it. Instead, take out a piece and put it on a plate, close the box and put the box in the kitchen. Fix a salad or steamed vegetables to go with your piece of pizza. You will satisfy your hunger pangs equally as well with fewer calories.

Bags/boxes of snack foods (potato chips, crackers, nuts, etc): Avoid eating directly from a large open bag, can, tub, or box. Instead, check the serving size on the back and get that amount. Put your serving on a plate, and then put the bag (can, tub, or box) back in the cabinet.

Eat the designated amount and check yourself. Are you still hungry? If so, then you probably should make yourself a healthy mini-meal to better satisfy your hunger.

Leftovers: After dinner is served, put leftovers away immediately. Otherwise the sight of the food might prompt you to eat when you aren't hungry.

Small bites add up: even one bite of a casserole can give you 50 calories. Multiply that by 6 bites and you can see how that amount can equal the calories in an entire meal.

Buffets

While buffets can be a challenge for those who want to build a better body, they don't have to be if you have a plan.

Member Guide pg. 89

Leader Note:
Review the tips in this section and ask students to share their tips.

Here are some tips:

- Never go to the buffet hungry. Eat a high fiber fruit before you go, such as an apple, pear, or orange. That way, you will have some food in your stomach and your blood sugar will remain stable so that you can think clearly enough to make wise decisions about what to eat.

- If you are at a family event that features a buffet, don't take nibbles directly from the table. Fix a plate with a reasonable portion of food (minimizing servings of high fat, high sugar foods), sit down, and eat it slowly. Enjoy and participate in the conversations around you.

- Are you still hungry? Wait 10 more minutes to be sure. You can always go back for more. If you are still hungry, then only fix the amount that will satisfy the level of hunger that remains and enjoy it thoroughly.

- Always eat a large salad first in a restaurant buffet. Then you will be less hungry for the refined starches and desserts that you'll encounter afterward. But remember - go easy on the salad dressing, cheese, bacon bits, and croutons. These toppings can turn a healthy salad into a nutritional nightmare!

Stress Eating

**Member Guide
pg. 90**

Leader Note:
*Demonstrate
the Tension
Release
Exercise and
ask students to
follow along.*

Under stress, it is very easy to become vulnerable to bad habits. After all, your first instinct is to relieve the tension and bad habits are familiar and comfortable. Here are a few healthier techniques you can try to release tension rather than turning to food:

Tension Release Exercise

Find a quiet, comfortable place free from distractions. The location can be on your bed, on the carpet, or in your favorite chair. Close your eyes and breathe deeply.

Begin by inhaling and tensing your feet for five seconds; exhale slowly, releasing the tension. Next, tense the muscles in your lower legs for five seconds and inhale; let them relax while exhaling slowly. Continue the pattern, moving up your body. Let your muscles of your face be the last group to tense and release. Allow tension to completely drain away from each muscle group with every exhalation.

The 3/4/5 Breathing Exercise

Another relaxation exercise to try is the 3/4/5 breathing exercise, which involves focusing on your breathing without the muscle tensing action. Again, you will need to steal away to a quiet, comfortable place. For a minute or two, focus on your breath going in and going out.

Then, do the following:

1. Inhale slowly for a count of three.

2. Hold the breath for a count of four.

3. Exhale slowly for a count of five.

4. Repeat five times.

Music Therapy

A highly effective means to relax is music therapy. The most effective music styles for this purpose are praise and worship music, classical, and modern instrumental.

Other types of music that assist in relaxation are recorded nature sounds. Tapes that feature sounds like ocean waves or rain can be extremely calming. Or better yet, you can experience these pleasures in person.

Stress Eating, continued

Member Guide pg. 91

Returning to Nature

Find the nearest park or nature preserve near you and take a walk, paying attention to the sounds of birds or running streams. Pretend to be a child again and glory in the details you experience: the smell of fresh pine, the intricacies and varieties of the leaves on the trees, and the snapping of twigs under your feet. The beauty and power of nature is healing and helps to reaffirm your connection to your Creator.

Sleep and rest

If you aren't allowing yourself enough time to sleep and rest, you will not be able to function and enjoy life to its fullest. Each day is precious; make sure that you recharge those batteries every day so that you stay alert and ready to handle challenges with grace and creativity. Adequate sleep is also essential to help your body drop excess weight more readily.

Check out the National Sleep Foundation at http://www.sleepfoundation.org for guidance if you are having problems getting adequate sleep.

Food Pushing Relatives

Leader Note: Ask students if they have any food pushing relatives – ask them not to give names to protect the guilty!

If you have a relative or friend who constantly offers you unhealthy, but tempting food, then just realize that this person probably thinks that food equals love. She believes she is showing you her love by feeding you. So occasional acceptance of the gesture might be wise, but most often you can politely decline, expressing much gratitude for the loving offer.

When these well-meaning people place such food in front of you after you have eaten your quota, you might can say, "Everything was so wonderful! I love your food but I honestly couldn't eat another bite."

If someone continues to insist, you can say, "You know, I need to take a break. I may have some later." Be kind, but be firm. If she is persistent, continue to decline - like a broken record, if necessary. Eventually, the person will get the message.

Losing Motivation

Member Guide pg. 92

To avoid losing your motivation with your weight loss goals, then give yourself regular "CPR." In this case, CPR stands for Consistency, Passion, and Rewards.

- Consistency means practicing your new habits until they start to feel comfortable. When that happens, you know that your brain is starting to make the habits automatic so that they are easy to maintain.

  Consistency moves your habits into your *procedural memory,* which is the same part of your memory that stores procedures like 'how to brush your teeth,' 'how to ride a bike' or 'how to drive to work'. You don't have to teach yourself these things over and over – you've done them so much that you don't have to think about them anymore!

  Likewise, when you practice healthy habits over and over, eventually you won't have to think about them anymore. Like the Nike slogan, you'll "Just do it".

- Passion comes from the belief that you can have the body that you deserve and that you are willing to do what it takes to get it.

  You can inflame a passion for your goal by visualizing it as if you have already achieved it. Do this at least twice a day, preferably while you are exercising. Make the experience as vivid as you can. Experience the pleasure and satisfaction you will have once you reach your goal. This will keep you inspired until your dream is made reality.

- Reward yourself with a nonfood item every time you practice a healthy habit. You want to reinforce both the behaviors that will get you results as well as the results themselves. Your reward could be as simple as a hug, pat on the back, or hot bubble bath. Larger rewards could include a relaxation CD, taking in a movie, or getting a massage.

The more pleasure you associate with your new habits, the more you will want to repeat them. This will also lead to more discipline and make it likely that you will keep these habits (and your new healthier body) for life.

Member Guide pg. 93

Leader Note: *Review the tips in this section and ask students to share their tips.*

The importance of passing on good habits to children is a special responsibility. Studies repeatedly show that overweight children almost always have at least one parent who is overweight. While heredity does play a part, the greater factor is that children tend to eat what their parents eat. Try easing your family into a healthier diet with the following tips:

- Don't bring unhealthy food choices into the house. As long as these foods are in the house, the family will probably choose to eat those instead of healthy foods. They may protest at first - when the usual snack items are discovered missing, but will be much happier once they begin to enjoy a lifestyle of nutritious eating, gaining energy, and looking better.

   Alternatively, you can take the "weaning" approach by selecting one unhealthy snack item to bring into the house. Make it the smallest bag/box you can buy. When it's gone, it's gone. Do this a time or two and then stop buying the snack completely.

- Keep fruits and vegetables readily available. Keep a fruit bowl on the kitchen table or counter filled with fruits your family likes. Peaches, nectarines, and bananas are usually popular with children. You can also keep a prepared vegetable plate of carrots, celery, and tomato slices in the refrigerator with low fat dip.

- Sneak vegetables into the foods you cook. Add extra vegetables to spaghetti sauce, soups, stews, and casseroles. Add fruit to yogurt or cereal. Also buy the "chunky" varieties of salsa and spaghetti sauce to get extra vegetable servings. Use leftover vegetables in a stir fry or salad.

- Find lower fat, lower calorie versions of your favorite recipes on the Internet. Experts agree that most families eat the same 5-7 meals regularly every month. If you can either find a healthier version of the meal to prepare or make a tasty substitution, then you will make staying healthy easier.

- You can also search for delicious ways to prepare fruits and vegetables. There are some vegetable recipes in the back of this book. You can also get more recipes at www.morematters.org.

Emotional Eating

Member Guide pg. 94

For emotional eating, use your journal to help you determine what emotions are driving your behavior.

Think about the following questions when you eat:

- Were you hungry?

- What was the emotion if you weren't hungry?

- Did you eat fast or slow?

- Did you eat when you were satisfied or past full?

Were you hungry?

This question was designed to get you to start being aware of your body's signals. Typical signs of hunger are slight discomfort in your stomach, stomach growling, low energy, etc. This means that your body actually needs food. When you look at your journal, how often did you eat when you were not hungry? Make a note of it.

What was the emotion if not hungry?

This is critical. What were the emotions that you felt most often when you were driven to eat...were you bored, angry, lonely, tired, or some other emotion? Actually take an honest look at what's really going on. This is what you need to be dealing with. Make a note of the emotions that seem to drive your behavior most often.

Did you eat fast or slow?

Most people who have emotional eating issues generally eat quite fast. They don't really taste and enjoy their food. The goal is to eat quickly until they can't eat anymore. Then a feeling of numbness sets in. When you eat emotionally, you are trying to 'pacify' yourself. Think of a baby pacifier. When a baby is cranky, you often stick a pacifier in her mouth to calm her down. It works temporarily, until the next go-around.

That's the way food is. You might eat to pacify yourself, which keeps you from dealing with the real issues in your life for a time. However, the problems never go away with food. They are only buried under them.

You need the courage to confront the issues in your life head-on and come up with a specific plan for dealing with them. All the while, seek support from others and wisdom from God in how to best handle these problems.

Emotional Eating, continued

Did you eat until you were satisfied or past full?

In emotional eating patterns, there is a compulsion to finish everything on your plate whether your body has had enough or not. Again, it is an attempt to pacify, to keep eating until the numbness sets in.

Member Guide pg. 95

An emergency technique:

The next time you are tempted to eat when you are not hungry, just pause. Drink a glass of water and wait for 10 minutes. During that time, pray silently with the following scripture in mind:

Romans 14:17: "For the kingdom of God is not eating and drinking, but righteousness and peace and joy in the Holy Spirit."

Ask God to fill you with His peace and joy in that moment. Breathe slowly, and deeply, keeping your mind focused on that scripture.

Don't get distressed if the urge to eat during the 10 minutes comes up. Just refocus on your breathing and on the scripture.

After 10 minutes, ask yourself...do you still want to eat? Just by pausing and shifting your focus, you'll find that you don't want to eat any longer.

The ultimate goal when you are faced with overwhelming, negative emotions is to anchor yourself in God first - rather than turning to food.

As mentioned previously, your goal is to move your new habits into your procedural memory by consistent practice so that you don't have to think about them any longer.

Use this new procedure to handle emotional eating urges. Practice it over and over and soon it will become a habit that will serve you better.

My Test Action Plan

Member Guide pg. 96 (students will complete this for homework)

Potential tests	Ways I can handle them

Week 7 Homework Instructions

 Leader Note: Explain the activities for homework to be completed <u>before</u> Week 8's class

Read 1 Corinthians 10:13 and answer the following question.

1. Is there any temptation that you've had that no one else has ever had?

    _____

    _____

2. What does the scripture say about God's character?

    _____

    _____

3. How does God demonstrate his faithfulness in temptations?

    _____

    _____

5. How can you use this information the next time you face a temptation?

    _____

    _____

    _____

Walk it Out Activities:

*   Memorize next week's focus scripture.
*   Review the tests that have been outlined in the lesson and place a checkmark by the tests that you have faced before or those you might face in the future.
*   Complete the Test Action plan on the previous page to begin thinking of ways you can deal with the tests that you will likely face in implementing your weight loss plan. Write down any tests that you faced this week in your journal and how you handled them. If you didn't handle your challenges as well as you liked, write down what you will do differently next time.

Week 8: Putting it All Together

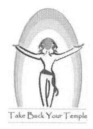

Take Back Your Temple

Week 8 Focus Scripture:

Beloved, I pray that you may prosper in all things and be in health, just as your soul prospers.

- 3 John 1:2   (NKJV)

Lesson Goals

*Member Guide
pg. 99*

In this lesson, you will learn how to:

- Incorporating TBYT principles into your life
- Ways to ensure the weight you lose stays gone
- The one attitude you will need to succeed long term

*Lesson
Agenda*

*Quick
Overview*

- Welcome
- *Tense, Breathe, Jello Shake* exercise
- Recite this week's focus scripture
- Review the previous week's homework
- Review this week's lesson

Leader Lesson Agenda

- (5 minutes) *Open in prayer.*
- (5 minutes) *Tense, Breathe, Jello Shake exercise.*
- (5 minutes) *Welcome everyone to class and document attendance.*
- (10 minutes) *Ask each person to recite this week's focus scripture.*
- (20 minutes) *Review the previous week's homework – answers follow on the next page.*
- (10 minutes) *Journal review* – Ask each person to turn in their Healthy Habits journals for review.

Ask the class to divide themselves into groups of 2 or 3. While you are reviewing the journals, ask each group to discuss the following question: *"What has been your biggest test in practicing a healthy lifestyle? What is your plan for staying on track going forward?"*

After you have checked the journals, return them to their owners.

- (20 minutes) *Review this week's lesson and discuss*
- (30 minutes) *Ask if person to share the results they have had as a result of participating in the TBYT study and lessons learned.*
- (5 minutes) *Close in prayer and thank students for their participation. Issue completion certificates.*

Week 7 Homework – Answers

Leader Note: Have homework group discussion, asking for feedback for each question.

Read 1 Corinthians 10:13 and answer the following question.

1. Is there any temptation that you've had that no one else has ever had?

   - *Ask 1-2 students to contribute to this discussion.*

2. What does the scripture say about God's character?

   God is faithful

3. How does God demonstrate his faithfulness in temptations?

   With temptations He makes a way of escape so that we can bear them.

4. How can you use this information the next time you face a temptation?

   - *Ask 1-2 students to contribute to this discussion.*

Lesson Introduction

Member Guide pg. 100

The rallying cry for this section is, "You took it back; don't give it back!" You've been given a lot of information, but it's up to you to take what applies to your specific needs, and use your creativity to incorporate it into the way you live. Strive from this day forward to walk in the abundant life God has promised to those who seek and follow Him.

Remember that it will simply be one day and one choice at a time. Victory will come when all is said and done!

Keep in mind the simple way business philosopher Jim Rohn defines the difference between success and failure:

- Failure = a few errors in judgment practiced every day
- Success = a few simple disciplines practiced every day

The key to both of these conditions is the phrase *'practiced every day.'* It is that little extra effort you make every day to get healthy that ultimately determines if you'll succeed or not on your weight loss quest and enjoy the spoils of victory for a lifetime.

This lesson gives you a few tips on staying committed to staying healthy.

The Power of Influence

A famous speaker once said that if you want to know where you are headed, check out your friends. His warning was that wherever they are is where you are likely to be (or end up). Human beings thrive on relationships; we can influence others and be influenced by them.

To ensure that your health influences are positive, you need a few friends who are in good shape and are using healthy means to stay that way. You might join a walking group or a nutrition class to that you can hang out with others like you are now. You can even continue meeting with the members of your class as ongoing support!

Let your health-conscious friends spur you on to greater levels of health. You will also have the opportunity to change their lives for the better as well by sharing your inspirational story. It's a win/win situation all around!

124

A Personal Story: A Little Extra Effort

Let's end our time together with a special story. It is actually true and happened to Kim Taylor, the creator of TBYT, when she was a high school senior. This experience shaped her entire life.

When she was in high school, she took a specialized literature class. It was quite a large class, maybe 30 students in all. The teacher decided to give the students an assignment for extra credit. They had three choices as to which assignment to do:

Member Guide pg. 101

- Memorize and recite a 16-line poem to receive an 'A' grade
- Memorize and recite a 12-line poem to receive a 'B' grade
- Memorize and recite a 4-line poem to receive a 'D' grade

The teacher gave the students a week to fulfill the assignment. On the appointed date, she asked each student to stand up and recite his or her chosen poem. Out of the 30 students, can you guess how many chose to do the 'A' poem? One student. Can you guess how many students chose to do the 'B' poem? One student.

The other *28 students* chose to do the 'D' poem assignment.

That experience has stayed with Kim because she was the only student who chose to do the 'A' poem. After she finished reciting it, the other students applauded, but the experience puzzled her. Why had the other students chosen to do only the minimum? The reward was obvious. Maybe they looked at the 16 lines and decided that the task was too big and too hard.

But Kim discovered the task wasn't hard at all. She decided not to focus on learning all 16 lines at once - but on pacing herself. She memorized 3-4 lines each day. Then when the assignment was due, she had accumulated all 16 lines of the poem in her mind, so reciting them to the class was not difficult at all! She achieved her with simple commitment to practicing small steps every day.

Right now, you might be looking at your health goals and having a hard time believing they will come to pass. Take the lessons Kim learned from her high school assignment and apply it to your weight challenges. If you merely focus on making positive day-to-day choices, they will gradually add up and you too can accomplish the highest level of achievement that you could dream.

The Ultimate Success Secret

Member Guide pg. 102

All it takes is a little extra effort on your part to seek God's direction and renew your mind daily according His word and His will. This fabulous formula will make all the difference in your weight, your health, and your life – both temporally and eternally!

To have the power to do the right thing even when it is challenging, anchor yourself in God's love every day through prayer, praise, worship, and study of the Word. Generate that faith shield first thing in the morning. God is your banner, your strength, and your stronghold. You cannot win this challenge without Him.

We pray that you will experience **all** of the goodness that God has laid up for you and that you will stand before Him at the end of your life and have Him say to you: "Well done, thy good and faithful servant. Enter into the joy of your Lord."

Appendix

Using Food to Balance Your Mood

Do you experience stress, anxiety, depression, irritability, and emotional upsets frequently? If your diet consists mostly of sugar, high fat, and refined starchy food (the starches that have had the bran removed), it is likely these foods are interfering with your brain function.

To maintain emotional stability, the brain must maintain a delicate balance between three chemicals:

- Glucose, maintains your blood sugar levels
- Serotonin, a neurotransmitter associated with feelings of calm and relaxation
- Beta-endorphin, the body's natural pain relievers

Eating too many processed foods disrupt that balance. To get out of the cycle, you must eat foods that stabilize the production of these chemicals to return the brain to balance. Which foods? These would be foods high in 'B' and 'C' vitamins and the mineral Zinc. You also need foods high in fiber.

As you might have guessed, most of these vitamins and minerals you need to maintain brain balance are found in fruits and vegetables. In the general eating pattern I've given you, it was also recommended that you include healthy fats in your diet to help increase your food satisfaction level. Such fats include: olive oil, canola oil, flax seed oil, almonds and other nuts, as well as cold water fish like wild Atlantic salmon.

Because your body's needs may change on a daily basis, pay close attention to how you feel with this new nutrition plan. Depending on how you feel, some days you may need to shift the balance to more lean protein, and some days you may need to favor more starchy food. In other words, you'll still eat the same amount of calories overall but the ratio of lean protein and starch will be different.

Some variations to try follow on the next page.

Mood: Having a short attention span, feeling sluggish, procrastinating a lot

- **Prescription:** Replace one of your portions of starchy vegetables/whole grain food in your diet for an extra portion of lean protein.

- **Why:** Increased 4-5 ounces of protein encourages the production of two brain chemicals (dopamine and norepinephrine) that keep you alert and focused.

Mood: Feeling stressed, overwhelmed, or stuck

- **Prescription:** Replace one of your portions of lean protein in your diet for an extra portion of a starchy vegetable or whole grain. Good choices for this purpose are sweet potatoes/yams or whole grain pasta.

- **Why:** These foods increase production of a neurotransmitter called serotonin, which increases feelings of calm and relaxation.

Health Tracking Log - Weekly

Date _____

Food category	Portions Eaten/Drank						
	S	**M**	**T**	**W**	**Th**	**F**	**Sa**
Water 8-12 cups per day, depending on your weight Water goal _____	☐☐ ☐☐ ☐☐ ☐☐ ☐☐ ☐☐	☐☐ ☐☐ ☐☐ ☐☐ ☐☐ ☐☐	☐☐ ☐☐ ☐☐ ☐☐ ☐☐ ☐☐	☐☐ ☐☐ ☐☐ ☐☐ ☐☐ ☐☐	☐☐ ☐☐ ☐☐ ☐☐ ☐☐ ☐☐	☐☐ ☐☐ ☐☐ ☐☐ ☐☐ ☐☐	☐☐ ☐☐ ☐☐ ☐☐ ☐☐ ☐☐
Fruits and Vegetables Vegetables: 5 portions/day Fruit: 2 portions/day	☐☐ ☐☐ ☐ ☐☐	☐☐ ☐☐ ☐ ☐☐	☐☐ ☐☐ ☐ ☐☐	☐☐ ☐☐ ☐ ☐☐	☐☐ ☐☐ ☐ ☐☐	☐☐ ☐☐ ☐ ☐☐	☐☐ ☐☐ ☐ ☐☐
Lean Protein 3-4 portions/day	☐☐☐ ☐	☐☐☐ ☐	☐☐☐ ☐	☐☐☐ ☐	☐☐☐ ☐	☐☐☐ ☐	☐☐☐ ☐
Whole grains/starchy vegetables 3 portions/day	☐☐ ☐	☐☐ ☐	☐☐ ☐	☐☐ ☐	☐☐ ☐	☐☐ ☐	☐☐ ☐
Healthy fats 1 portion/day	☐	☐	☐	☐	☐	☐	☐

Physical Activity Notes:

_____

_____

_____

Slimming Meal Tips

To make it easier for you to lose weight, here are some meal ideas for breakfast, lunch and dinner.

Breakfast Ideas

Bacon and eggs

> 1 scrambled egg
> 2 strips of turkey bacon
> ½ whole wheat bagel
> 1 orange

Cereal

> 1 cup 1% milk
> ¾ cup whole grain cereal
> 1 medium banana

Breakfast Bar (great on-the-go option)

> 1 high fiber breakfast bar (at least 5 grams of fiber and 5 grams of protein)
> 1 medium apple
> 1 8 oz carton of 1% or skim milk

Oatmeal

> 1 cup 1% milk
> ¾ cup cooked oatmeal
> 1 baked apple with cinnamon

Waffle

> 1 whole grain waffle
> ½ cup of fruit cocktail in its own juice
> ½ cup of vanilla yogurt

AM Snack Ideas

Each of the following snacks approximately 100 calories or less:

- A medium-sized apple
- A medium-sized orange
- A medium-sized banana
- ½ grapefruit
- ½ large pear
- 1 cup berries (blueberries, strawberries, raspberries, or blackberries)
- 3 prunes
- ¼ cup raisins

Lunch Ideas

Open-faced Chicken Sandwich

    3 ounces grilled chicken breast
½ whole grain sandwich roll
1 slice lettuce, tomato, and onion
1 tbsp ketchup and mustard
1 cup of tomato, onion, and cucumber salad (made with 1 TBSP light Italian dressing)

Pasta Salad

    2 ounces of turkey ham
1 ounce of mozzarella cheese
1 red tomato, chopped
½ cup whole grain rotini or spiral pasta
1 tbsp light Balsamic vinaigrette dressing

        Mix all ingredients above and chill.

Serve over 1 cup mixed salad greens

Turkey Wrap

    3 ounces of roast turkey
Chopped tomato, lettuce, and onion
1 whole grain tortilla
1 tbsp light honey mustard dressing

Top the whole grain tortilla with the roast turkey, chopped vegetables, and dressing.

    1 cup roasted zucchini, squash, onions, and red pepper

Grilled Salmon

    3 ounces of grilled Salmon
1 small corn on the cob
1 cup of turnip greens

Soup

    1 cup of tomato or vegetable soup
2 ounces of cheddar or mozzarella cheese
1 cup steamed green beans

Chili

    ½ cup of black bean chili
½ cup of corn
1 cup of steamed broccoli/carrot mix

P.M. Snack Ideas

Each of these snacks has approximately 150 calories or less:

½ cup of pistachio nuts
1 oz roasted almonds (about 22 nuts)
1 oz walnuts
16 bittersweet chocolate chips

1 oz cashews (about 18 nuts)
1 oz roasted peanuts (about 25 nuts)
¼ cup sunflower seeds

Dinner Ideas

Spaghetti

> ½ cup of spaghetti with meat sauce
> ½ cup whole wheat spaghetti
> ½ cup steamed squash
> 1 cup of zucchini

Grilled Chicken

> 3 ounces of grilled chicken
> ½ cup of brown rice
> 1 cup of turnip greens
> ½ cup of roasted red peppers

Open-faced Turkey Burger

> 3 ounces broiled turkey burger patty
> ½ whole grain sandwich roll
> 1 slice lettuce, tomato, and onion
> ½ c. sautéed green peppers and
> mushrooms
> 1 tbsp ketchup and mustard
>
> 1 cup of mixed green salad with 1 Tbsp
> Italian dressing

Oven-fried fish

> 3 ounces of oven fried Whiting
> 1 small sweet potato
> 1 cup of spinach
> ½ cup of carrots

Soup

> 1/2 cup of lentil soup
> 1 small whole wheat roll
> 1 cup steamed green beans
> ½ cup of sautéed mushrooms

Beef or Chicken Fajitas

> ½ cup of beef or chicken fajita
> seasoned meat
> 1 whole wheat tortilla
> ½ cup of sautéed onion and pepper
> strips
> ¼ cup of salsa
> 1 cup of steamed broccoli/carrot mix

Making Meals Convenient and Delicious

When it comes to preparing meals and snacks, simple is better. Here are a few tips that can help you make eating healthy convenient for yourself.

Keep Fruit in Sight

Another tip is to keep a fruit bowl on the counter or dining room table. Keeping it within sight and easy reach makes it more likely you will eat them.

For your servings, select the whole fruit rather than juices whenever possible. Whole fruit contains fiber, which helps you feel satisfied on fewer calories. For example: 2/3 of a cup of orange juice contains 85 calories while a medium orange has about 65 calories.

You also want to select the whole fruit rather than dried pieces most often. Because dried fruit has had its water removed, its calories are more concentrated when compared to the original fruit. For example, a cup of grapes is about 100 calories. But it only takes ¼ cup of raisins to get 100 calories. The grapes would certainly be more satisfying ultimately.

*Juicy fruit gives you a bigger size snack than the same fruit dried—for the same number of calories.

Another alternative to whole fruit is to keep several cans of fruit in its own juice around to make it easier to acquire enough fruit servings.

Cook in Batches

Be sure that you have plenty of fruits, vegetables, whole grains, and lean protein in your home. One thing that helps me out is to batch cook on Saturdays. I cook vegetables, broil chicken breasts, oven-fried fish, and bake sweet potatoes. Then I freeze it all in smaller containers. That way, when I'm busy during the week, I just take the prepared healthy foods out of the freezer and put them together for a quick, reheated meal.

Buy Quick Change Ingredients

My favorite foods to buy are those that can be used in different types of meals. Here are some of my favorite quick change ingredients:

Chicken

- Roast it whole, use in salad, wraps, fajitas

Whole Wheat Tortillas

- Use them for sandwich wraps, burritos, fajitas or cut into triangles and bake into chips to use with salsa for snacks or sprinkle with cinnamon and brown sugar as a sweet treat.

Ground Beef

- Use for chili, spaghetti, hobo dinner (ground beef patty topped with onions, garlic, carrots, and sweet potatoes, wrapped in foil and baked at 350 degrees for about 30 minutes)

Tip: To lower the fat in ground beef, do the following:

Buy ground beef or ground turkey, but brown it and drain off the excess fat. Rinse the cooked beef with hot water, drain again, and then blot the crumbles lightly with white paper towels. This procedure reduces the fat by 50%.

Brown Rice

- Prepare plain, as a pilaf (with chicken broth, onion, garlic, frozen peas and carrots), or unfried rice (TBSP of oil, egg, rice, green onions, TBSP light soy sauce, frozen peas and carrots)

Eggs

- Prepare as scrambled or as an omelet (use 3 eggs, but remove 2 of the yolks) or use in unfried rice

Beans

- Use them in burritos, chili, soups, and salads

Make Quick Change Salads

I learned this trick from a cookbook I bought years ago: buy seven salad ingredients that you can mix and match for variety.

Here are the seven ingredients

- 1 head of red cabbage
- 2 bags of mixed greens
- 3 red onions
- 4 cucumbers
- 5 carrots
- 6 plum tomatoes
- Low fat vinaigrette dressing

Salad #1: Marinated greens

    2 cups of mixed greens marinated with ¼ cup of vinaigrette

Salad #2: Cucumber, tomato, and onion

    Combine 1 peeled sliced cucumber, 1 plum tomato, and ½ sliced red onion with ¼ cup of vinaigrette

Salad #3: Mixed greens and tomato

    Combine 1 cup of mixed greens and 1 plum tomato with ¼ cup of vinaigrette

Salad #4: Marinated tomatoes

    Combine 2 sliced plum tomatoes and ½ cup of chopped red onion with ¼ c of vinaigrette

Salad #5: Marinated cucumbers and onion

    Combine 1 peeled sliced cucumber and ½ sliced red onion with ¼ cup of vinaigrette

Salad #6: Coleslaw

    Combine 2 cups of shredded cabbage with 1 cup of shredded carrots and ½ chopped red onion with ¼ cup of vinaigrette

Salad #7: Mixed salad

Combine 3 cups of mixed greens, 1 cup shredded red cabbage, 2 peeled sliced cucumbers, ½ cup of chopped onion, 2 sliced plum tomatoes, 1 cup sliced carrots, and ½ cup of vinaigrette

Use Frozen Vegetables to Save Time

While fresh vegetables are best, frozen vegetables can be more convenient. They are generally cheaper too, especially if you find them on sale.

A typical 16 ounce bag of frozen vegetables contains 5 portions of vegetables, which is the amount that you will be eating per day. Prepare your vegetables first thing in the morning. Mix ½ cup of water and 1 tbsp. of dry soup mix (herb and garlic, onion and mushroom, and golden onion are my favorites). You can also use ½ cup of low sodium chicken and vegetable broth to cook your vegetables.

Pour the mixture into a saucepan and put in the package of frozen vegetables. Bring the mixture to a boil and then turn down the heat to low. Then cover the pan with a lid and cook the veggies for 8-10 minutes. You can either eat the vegetables warm or add fresh tomato, onion, mushroom, or cucumber to the vegetables with some light Balsamic vinegrette dressing and spices and chill to make a salad. Quick, easy, and tasty!

Roast Vegetables for Maximum Flavor

Another favorite way to cook vegetables is to roast them. Roasting vegetables seems to bring out their sweetness and flavor. Here is a favorite roasted vegetables recipe.

Ingredients

½ red pepper, cut into large pieces
1 large zucchini, sliced
2 large yellow squash, sliced
1 c. sliced mushrooms
½ medium red onion, sliced
5 cloves garlic
2 tbsp. of light balsamic vinaigrette dressing

Directions

Preheat the oven to 375 degrees. Spray a baking pan lightly with olive oil. Place all of the vegetables in the pan and bake for 10 minutes (edges of the vegetables should be lightly browned). Remove the pan from the oven and turn the vegetables over so that the other side of them is browned. Bake the vegetables for another 5-10 minutes.

Remove the pan from the oven. Place the roasted cloves of garlic in a large bowl. Mash the cloves of garlic together. Add the balsamic vinaigrette dressing. Mix the dressing and garlic together. Add the remainder of the vegetables and toss the mixture together.

These vegetables are delicious warm or cold.

Make Vegetable Soup in the Crockpot

Another great way to get your vegetable servings is to make a large pot of vegetable soup. To make it easier, use a crockpot because you can put the ingredients in a pot and let it cook while you go on to other things.

Here is my favorite recipe for spicy crockpot vegetable soup. I use frozen vegetables for convenience.

Ingredients

1 medium onion, chopped
1 green pepper, chopped
1/2 head of cabbage, chopped
16 ounce package of frozen mixed vegetables
1 can of stewed tomatoes, drained
1 teaspoon thyme
1 tbsp of Cajun seasoning
2 cloves garlic, minced
1 cup reduced fat chicken broth
2 cups of tomato juice
1 packet of dry onion soup mix

Directions

Combine all ingredients in a large crockpot. Set the crockpot on low and cook for 6-8 hours.

Oven fry meats

In the Southern U.S., deep frying is second nature. If you grew up with fried chicken and fried fish, it may be difficult to grow accustomed to baked chicken and fish.

To bridge the gap, you can fry chicken and fish in the oven. Here is a recipe for oven fried fish. If you are short on time, you can substitute prepared seafood coating for the first four ingredients.

Ingredients

3/4 c. cornmeal
1 tsp. pepper
1 tsp. garlic powder
1 tsp. Cajun spice
1 egg lightly beaten
2 Tbsp. water
2 Tbsp. lemon juice
1 lb. fish fillets (such as whitefish or Alaskan Pollack)
Vegetable oil spray

Directions

Preheat oven to 425 degrees. Spray flat baking pan with vegetable oil spray. Mix cornmeal, pepper, garlic powder, and Cajun spice in a large flat dish or plate. Mix egg and water together. Rinse fish and pat dry; sprinkle each filet with lemon juice and dip in egg mixture. Coat the fish with cornmeal mixture and place in pan in single layer. Spray fillets lightly with vegetable oil spray. Bake for 15 minutes and then turn. Bake for another 10 minutes or until fish flakes easily with a fork. Serves four.

A Final Word on Eating Healthy

Whenever possible, avoid bringing the high fat, high sugar items into your home. If you bring the unhealthier items in and force yourself to choose between them versus more nutritious food, you will likely go for the fatty items because they are the most familiar. So make it easier on yourself by keeping healthy foods on hand and the junk out of stock!

Overcoming Barriers to Exercise

If you've been having difficulty starting or sticking to an exercise program, help is here! According to a U.S. Department of Health and Human Service (USDHHS) report, the 10 most common barriers adults face to being physically active are as follows:

- Do not have enough time to exercise
- Inconvenient to exercise
- Lack of self-motivation
- Do not find exercise enjoyable
- Find exercise boring
- Low confidence in ability to be physically active
- Fear of being injured or a recent injury
- Lack of ability to set goals and stay on track
- Lack of encouragement, support, or companionship from family and friends
- Do not have parks, sidewalks, bicycle trails, or safe and pleasant walking paths convenient to their homes or offices.

And here is an 11th barrier often heard from women:

- The sweat makes my hair nappy or frizzy, and my body feel dirty and smelly

The following are the USDHHS suggestions for overcoming the top 10 barriers.

Suggestions for Overcoming Physical Activity Barriers

Lack of time	Identify available time slots by monitoring your daily activities for one week. Identify at least three 15-minute time slots you could use for physical activity each day.
	Add physical activity to your daily routine. For example, walk or ride your bike to work or shopping, organize school activities around physical activity, walk the dog, exercise while you watch TV, park farther away from your destination, etc.
	Make time for physical activity. For example, walk, jog, or swim during your lunch hour, or take fitness breaks instead of coffee breaks.
	Select activities requiring minimal time, such as walking, jogging, or stair-climbing.
Lack of motivation	Plan ahead. Make physical activity a regular part of your daily or weekly schedule and write it on your calendar.

Invite a friend to exercise with you on a regular basis and write it on both your calendars.

Join an exercise group or class.

Lack of energy

Schedule physical activity for times in the day or week when you feel energetic.

Convince yourself that if you give it a chance, physical activity will increase your energy level; then, try it.

Fear of injury

Learn how to warm up and cool down to prevent injury.

Learn how to exercise appropriately considering your age, fitness level, skill level, and health status.

Choose activities involving minimum risk.

Lack of skill

Select activities requiring no new skills, such as walking, climbing stairs, or jogging.

Exercise with friends who are at the same skill level as you are.

Find a friend who is willing to teach you some new skills.

Take a class to develop new skills.

Lack of resources

Select activities that require minimal facilities or equipment, such as walking, jogging, jumping rope, or calisthenics.

Identify inexpensive, convenient resources available in your community (community education programs, park and recreation programs, worksite programs, etc.).

Weather conditions

Develop a set of regular activities that are always available regardless of weather (indoor cycling, aerobic dance, indoor swimming, calisthenics, stair climbing, rope skipping, mall walking, dancing, gymnasium games, etc.)

Look on outdoor activities that depend on weather conditions (cross-country skiing, outdoor swimming, outdoor tennis, etc.) as "bonuses"-extra activities possible when weather and circumstances permit.

Travel

Put a jump rope in your suitcase and use it - wearing supportive athletic shoes.

Walk the halls and climb the stairs in hotels. Stay in places with swimming pools or exercise facilities.

Join the YMCA or YWCA (ask about their reciprocal membership agreement).

Visit the local shopping mall and walk for half an hour or more as you window shop.

Bring a small tape recorder and your favorite aerobic exercise tape.

Family obligations   Trade babysitting time with a friend, neighbor, or family member who also has small children.

Exercise with the kids: go for a walk together, play tag or other running games, get an aerobic dance or exercise tape for kids (there are several on the market) and exercise together. You can spend time together and still get your exercise.

Hire a babysitter and look at the cost as a worthwhile investment in your physical and mental health.

Jump rope, do calisthenics, ride a stationary bicycle, or use other home gymnasium equipment while the kids are busy playing or sleeping.

Try to exercise when the kids are not around (e.g., during school hours or their nap time).

Encourage exercise facilities to provide child care services.

Retirement years   Look upon your retirement as an opportunity to become more active instead of less. Spend more time gardening, walking the dog, and playing with your grandchildren. Children with short legs and grandparents with slower gaits are often great walking partners.

Learn a new skill that's always interested you, such as ballroom dancing, square dancing, or swimming (great for folks with limited mobility).

Now that you have the time, make regular physical activity a part of every day. Go for a walk every morning or every evening before dinner. Treat yourself to an exercycle and ride every day while reading a favorite book or magazine, or watching a wholesome TV show.

Social influence   Explain your interest in physical activity to friends and family and ask them to support your efforts.

Invite friends and family members to exercise with you. Plan social activities involving exercise.

Develop new friendships with physically active people. Join a group, such as the YMCA or a hiking club.

Content for 'Suggestion for overcoming barriers' taken from *Promoting Physical Activity: A Guide for Community Action* (USDHHS, 1999).

As for the 11th barrier, here are some ideas to keep your hair looking good and your body fresh when you exercise:

- Keep your hair pulled away from your face and neck when you exercise.
- Consider blunt cuts or bobs since these haircuts keep their shape after exercise.
- Natural hair styles like braids are also convenient and stay in place after exercise.
- Keep your hair well conditioned and the ends trimmed regularly.
- If swimming is your primary exercise, always wear a cap to protect your hair from the effects of chlorine.
- To smooth the edges of your hairline after your workout, apply gel or cream to the area and smooth it down. Tie a scarf to cover the hairline and leave it on for 15 minutes. When you remove the scarf, your hairline should be smooth.
- To quick set your hair after a workout, try applying some wrapping lotion to the ends, cover with end papers and set it on rollers.
- A body remedy: At home wear old t-shirts or workout clothes during exercise and shower/deodorize before changing into clean ones. Away from home, quickly sponge bathe and dry your sweaty areas in a restroom and apply body powder that you brought along. Voila'! You're all fresh again!

20084241R00082

Printed in Poland
by Amazon Fulfillment
Poland Sp. z o.o., Wrocław